P9-BYN-634

THE SUCCESSFUL
MEDICAL STUDENT

Achieving Your Full Potential

IMPORTANT NOTICE

Because new research and clinical practice often lead to changes in treatment and drug dosages, readers should confirm the information presented in this book using other sources. The authors, the publisher, and the editors of this work have been careful to ensure that the information presented is accurate and conforms to accepted practices at the time of publication. Nevertheless, the possibility of human error, as well as new findings in the medical sciences, requires that the author, the publisher, and the editors of this work do not warrant that the information contained herein is accurate or complete in every respect.

THE SUCCESSFUL MEDICAL STUDENT

Achieving Your Full Potential

John R. Thornborough, Ph.D.
Mount Sinai School of Medicine
of The City University of New York

Hilary J. Schmidt, Ph.D.
State University of New York
Health Science Center at Brooklyn

**ILOC, Inc.
Publishers**

New York
Granville, Ohio

THE SUCCESSFUL MEDICAL STUDENT
Achieving Your Full Potential

Copyright © 1993 by The Upjohn Company. All rights reserved. Printed in the United States of America. No part of this publication may be reproduced in any form without the prior written permission of The Upjohn Company. Published by ILOC, Inc., 877 River Road, P.O. Box 232, Granville, OH 43023.

4 5 6 7 8 9 DOH 9 8 7 6

ISBN 1-882531-03-5

This book was set in Times Roman by ILOC, Inc.
The editor was Deborah Harvey.
The production supervisor was Diana Porter.
R.R. Donnelley & Sons was printer and binder.

Table of Contents

Preface   vii

1. What to Expect in Medical School
    The difference from college is quite significant so
you must anticipate some changes in your life-style.   1

2. A Time Line for the Next Five Years
    This chapter helps you plan for the major events
during your medical education.   9

3. Curricular Content
    Details of the medical school courses are pre-
sented in this chapter.   12

4. Financing Your Medical Education
    How to construct a budget to avoid unpleasant
financial surprises.   22

5. Basic Supplies for Your Study Desk
    You will need some essential items to be an
efficient and effective student.   35

6. What to Bring From College
    Certain facts, concepts, and skills that you learned
in college are needed in medical school.   41

7. Time Management
    How to organize and effectively use your time
even if you are married and have children.   49

8. Study Management
This chapter shows how to organize an efficient
learning process.   61

9. Getting the Most Out of Your Classes
Learn how to prepare for classes in advance and
become more efficient and effective.   72

10. Knowledge Organization
Determine the study method that best ensures
efficient learning and long-term memory.   81

11. Stress Management by Janice N. McLean, Ph.D.
This is a primer and pep talk to help you deal with
the stresses of medical school and beyond.   99

12. The Medical Specialties
In your fourth year you will choose one of these
specialties for your residency.   118

13. Medical Ethics by Rosamond Rhodes, Ph.D.
The complex moral issues in medicine for you to
consider.   136

14. A Summing Up of Ideas
Here is a list of helpful hints to help you over the
course of the next few years.   148

Preface

This book is for new medical students who are beginning a learning process that includes at least five years to become licensed to practice medicine, another one to four years of residency training, and, then, a lifetime of continued study while treating patients and/or doing research. It is a long and strenuous educational endeavor and can present many pitfalls along the way. This book was written to help you avoid these pitfalls.

Within this book we have included a great deal of information about your medical education. We describe what you may expect to find in your medical school curriculum and how that curriculum and its requirements are so different from what you have experienced in college. We provide some information on how to finance your education, list some basic items you will need for your place of study, and the skills and knowledge you should bring with you from college.

Most importantly, we will help you learn how to manage your time. It may seem obvious or trivial, but it is vital for you to realize that there are only 24 hours in each day and that a third to a half of them are absolutely committed to non-medical school activities. Thus, you must learn to budget your time if you are going to effectively and efficiently move through your medical education. If you learn to budget your time and study effectively, and we explain how this may be accomplished, not only will you be a successful medical student but also you will have spare time to actually enjoy the next four or five years.

Since medical school and the ensuing responsibilities of being a doctor are often very stressful and anxiety-provoking, we asked Janice N. McLean, a noted clinical psychologist, to write about those subjects. Her material will help you recognize your own stress and anxiety levels as well as offer tips on how to help yourself or to decide if professional help is needed.

A medical ethicist, Rosamond Rhodes, Ph.D., has written a chapter that will stimulate you to question and consider the ethical issues that frequently develop in the field of medicine. The issues both in medical school and medical practice are very complex and include such topics as rights and duties, justice, autonomy, truth-telling, and refusal of treatment. This list is not all inclusive, nor will all the issues be encountered by everyone; however, we believe they should be given careful consideration.

Finally, use and enjoy this little book. We are sure it will help you in many ways throughout your medical career.

John Thornborough
Hilary Schmidt

New York, NY, 1993

Chapter 1

What to Expect in Medical School

You are now in medical school – Congratulations on your acceptance into medical school! You have demonstrated your capabilities as an outstanding undergraduate and your medical school has selected you with confidence that you have the personal qualities and academic potential to become a good physician. However, success in an undergraduate program does not guarantee that you will achieve the same level of success in medical school. Imagine a college tennis player who has been a star in many intercollegiate competitions throughout his four years. When he graduates, he decides to enter the world of professional tennis. Would you be surprised if he was not seeded at Wimbledon, nor the winner of the U.S. Open? In this example, you easily recognize that there is a major difference between competition at the college and the professional level. You would not expect every college champion to excel in the professional tennis circuit. Moving from premedical studies in an undergraduate college to a professional medical school training program is analogous: quite simply, it is harder. This book offers many suggestions and guidelines to help you succeed on this higher level.

Most entering medical students were in the top 10% to 15% of their graduating class, but statistics guarantee that 50% will now end up in the bottom half of their medical school class. This is not as bad as it sounds; medical schools do not grade in the same way as undergraduate schools. The bottom 50% will not automatically "flunk being a doctor." In fact, some very good doctors will be from that bottom 50%.

Medical school presents an unparalleled challenge and for you to achieve your full potential you need to be aware of some of the basic differences between medical school and even the most rigorous premedical program. In addition, you should be aware of the typical and potentially detrimental misconceptions that many entering medical students have. An awareness of these issues will help you to design and implement a successful, high-yield study program.

What's the difference? – Medical school is different from college in three important ways: the volume of material, the level of detail, and the time constraints for study.

1. Volume – The sheer volume of material that must be mastered in medical school far exceeds any undergraduate demands. In most medical schools, the first two years cover gross anatomy, microanatomy, biochemistry, physiology, neuroscience, behavioral science, genetics, embryology, pathology, microbiology, immunology, pharmacology, and an introduction to clinical medicine. These courses provide a basic science foundation for the second two years, that typically cover medicine, surgery, pediatrics, obstetrics and gynecology, and psychiatry (see Chapter 3 for more details). The massive quantity of information that must be delivered requires an academic schedule filled with lectures, laboratories, conferences, and clinics that can occupy as many as seven hours a day, four to five days per week.

2. Detail – The detailed knowledge that is required of medical students is vast. You are expected to understand concepts and principles, and also their many accompanying specific facts and details. In Anatomy, for example, not only are you expected to understand how the origins and insertions of muscles predict their function, but you are also expected to know the exact name of each muscle, the bony processes and locations that demarcate the origins and insertions, the names of specific branches of nerves, and the blood supplies to that muscle. Likewise, in Biochemistry, you are expected to know how enzymes function in various chemical pathways, and also the exact name, chemical reaction, and role in a disease process for each involved enzyme.

Initially, many students underestimate the level of detail that is expected and at the time of the first examination, perceive the test to have focused on "picayune details." Don't forget that you are in training to become a physician, and the first two years are designed to provide you with the vocabulary and knowledge-base for the actual practice of medicine. It won't look good in the emergency room, if you need to refer to your anatomical atlas to figure out the pathway of a nerve that has been damaged, or to your biochemistry text to find out which enzymes might be involved in a disease process. Many exact facts need to be quickly and automatically accessible to you, and this training begins immediately.

You can become better prepared for the level of detail that is required by obtaining exams from previous years for each of your courses, and consulting with upper level students. Read through these exam questions before you even begin studying for a course to develop a sense of the content range, difficulty level, and amount of detail that you must achieve. This should help you focus your study in the most appropriate way, and ensure that you don't underestimate what is expected of you. In addition, memorization should be one of your daily study goals (see Chapter 8 for further discussion of this point).

3. Time constraints – It naturally follows that if you are expected to learn more information at a greater level of detail, within an academic schedule that requires you to be in classes most of the time, you are working under very tight time constraints. Going back to the tennis analogy, the pro returns the ball more frequently, at a higher speed, and to a wider range of locations. In order to "win" and master the medical school challenge, you must organize your time and approach your studies in a way that will ensure high efficiency and high productivity. Using the suggestions in *The Successful Medical Student* will help you do this.

Typical misconceptions – The first step to successful medical training is becoming aware of the demands; the next step is figuring out how to manage them.

1. Cramming – A potentially damaging misconception is that the study methods that worked well in an undergraduate environment will also be optimal in medical school. Some students may have been quite successful with cramming during college, but this approach is rarely effective in medical school. Cramming breeds confusion and does not lead to the level of mastery that is necessary. In addition, cramming does not yield long-term retention of information. At the end of the second year, students take a comprehensive national licensure examination covering all of the basic sciences, the United States Medical Licensing Examination (USMLE Step 1). It is important to have a study approach that will maximize long-term retention to ensure success on this examination as well as success later on in clinical practice.

2. Efficiency – A successful undergraduate approach that involved taking comprehensive notes from texts, integrating these with notes taken from lecture, and then developing summaries from the various sets of notes is just not efficient enough to work well in medical school. Any approach that does not involve highly organized time management, a commitment to keeping up to date, and active approaches to summarizing and organizing information is likely to require some adjustment. *The Successful Medical Student* will help you improve your study habits.

3. How other students study – Another potentially damaging misconception is that an approach that worked for an upper level student will also work for you. People are different in many ways. The texts, references, and methods that you find most useful will depend on your own background, personality, and cognitive skills.

Background – Some people have taken undergraduate courses that provided a solid foundation in the basic science subjects, while other students have little, if any, background in the same subjects. What works for an experienced student may be of little value to a novice and vice versa. For example, a basic reference may be of great help to the novice but of little use to a student with more experience. A student with a solid foundation in a subject may instead make more effective use of departmental handouts without the need for a basic reference text.

Personality – Some people are impulsive in their studies while others are more methodical and reflective. An impulsive student will likely recommend shorter, more succinct handouts and books that have an outline format. A more reflective student may prefer to study from textbooks, or references that are presented in paragraph format. In fact, neither approach by itself may be optimal. It is likely that a more impulsive student will neglect important details, and fail to take the time to reorganize information when necessary for effective long-term retention. On the other hand, the more reflective student may have great difficulty progressing at a pace that allows keeping up to date. We have made suggestions for study management that should guide you down the middle road that leads to learning detailed material quickly.

> See: Shain, D. *Study Skills and Test-Taking Strategies for Medical Students.* 1992. Springer-Verlag. New York Inc.: New York, N.Y. for a detailed treatment of individual differences in personal learning styles.

Cognitive Skills – People differ in their ability to learn various types of information. Some are very good at visual-spatial analysis, while others are not. Some are very good at mathematics, reading graphs, and analytical reasoning, while others are not. Some people have better reading skills than others. These kinds of differences in cognitive skills have a marked impact on the materials that are most useful to each individual. For example, someone who has strong visual analytical skills will learn anatomy with relative ease and will prefer to study from the atlas and cadaver. In contrast, someone with relatively poor visual analytical skills will struggle more and prefer anatomy texts that have more detailed written descriptions. You must use the method of study that works best for you.

Become aware of your own strengths and weaknesses – In summary, listen to but do not blindly accept the advice of other students. Rather, try to become aware of your own strengths and weaknesses and choose the texts and study methods that work most efficiently for you. The advice in the chapters that follow is based in part on research and principles of cognitive psychology (the science of learning, reasoning, memory, and problem solving) and in part on our years of experience in analyzing and evaluating the approaches of not only successful but also not-so-successful medical students.

Misconceptions About Medical School

1. Medical school won't be that different from under-graduate college.

2. My method of study from undergraduate college will be effective in medical school.

3. If a study approach works for someone else, it will undoubtedly work for me.

What it takes to achieve your full potential in medical school – There are many factors that will interact in complex ways to determine how successful you will be in medical school. Time organization; ability to manage lectures, texts, problem sets, and labs; implementation of active study techniques that yield long-term retention; performance on exams; and coping with stress all interact and influence each other. The diagram on the next page illustrates these interrelationships.

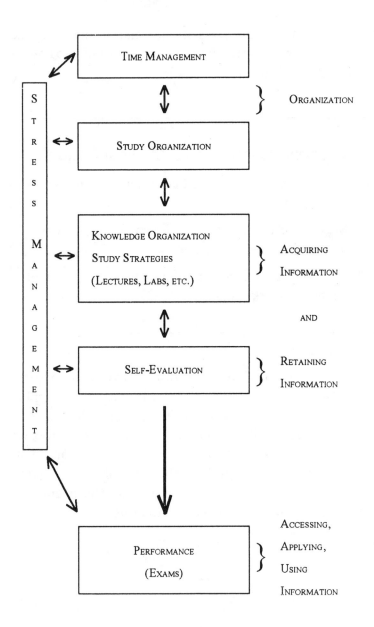

Chapter 2

A Time Line for the Next Five Years

Introduction – Over the next five years you will have many commitments and obligations to fulfill. It is very important that you not only remember them but also execute them in a timely manner. To aid you in this chore, we suggest that you use the following pages as the basis of a planning calendar. We have entered some of the known, important milestones and you should enter these and your own commitments into your master calendar as you become aware of them.

A brief note about money – Many of your obligations will involve the expenditure of money. For most medical students, money is tight and unexpected expenses are difficult to pay. We have marked with dollar signs those items on the time line that require money. In some cases we have estimated costs, but you should check these as the time draws near so that you will have an accurate idea of how much money you will need. (Chapter 4 contains ideas on how to budget your money.)

First year – This is a basic science year during which most of your time will be spent in the classroom. Enter on your calendar the dates of your tuition payments, activity fee, health insurance expenses, other insurance, rent and housing deposit, telephone and electric company deposit, equipment deposits, microscope rental, stethoscope and dissecting instrument purchase, and book expenses. Other important dates include deadlines for applications for summer employment, summer research, special summer courses, etc.

Second year – This is also a basic science year and much of your time will be in the classroom. During this year you may have Physical Diagnosis and will be expected to purchase various items of equipment. Check your school's schedule and requirements and be sure to budget for this large expense. Enter the dates of your tuition payments, activity fee, health insurance expenses, other insurance, rent, equipment deposits, and book expenses. Other important dates include deadlines for applications for USMLE Step 1, summer employment, summer research, special summer courses, etc.

> **March** – Application Deadline USMLE Step 1 $200.00

> **June** – First week: USMLE Step 1

Third year – This is your first clinical science year and you will spend most of your time interacting with patients. Be sure to schedule all of these sessions carefully. Most medical schools are very serious about your obligation to keep scheduled activities with patients. As before, enter the dates of your tuition payments, activity fee, health insurance expenses, other insurance costs, rent, equipment deposits, and book expenses. Other important dates include deadlines for applications for fourth-year electives within your own school and elsewhere, summer employment, summer research, special summer courses, etc.

> **January** – Application Deadline USMLE Step 2 $200.00

> **March/April** – USMLE Step 2

Fourth year – In your last year of medical school, you will spend the majority of your time taking electives as well as interviewing and applying for residency programs. Be sure to schedule all of these sessions carefully. You won't want to make a bad impression on the director of a residency program by missing an appointment. As before, enter the dates of your tuition payments, activity fee, health insurance expenses, other insurance costs, rent, and book expenses. Other important dates include deadlines for applications for fourth year electives both within your own school and elsewhere, residency program visits, application for the residency match, etc. Be sure to budget the cost of any electives out of town, cost of interviews, and travel and housing.

July – Last week: Student Agreements with the National Residency Match Program (NRMP) $$

August – Throughout the fall: Request information about residency programs

Last week: USMLE Step 2 (also next March)

October – The NRMP Directory of Programs is sent to applicants

November 1 – Dean's Letters for NRMP and specialty matching plans are mailed to applicant's programs

January – NRMP Rank Order List instructions and Directory Supplement are sent to participants

Mid: Results of the Ophthalmology Match announced

End: Results of the Otolaryngology Match announced

Late: Results of the Neurosurgery Match announced

February – Early: Results of the Neurology Match announced

Early: Results of the Urology Match announced

Last week: NRMP must receive Rank Order Lists

March – Third week: Results of the NRMP Match announced

Last week: USMLE Step 2

Chapter 3

Curricular Content

Introduction – The courses you take in medical school and the order in which you take them depends upon the curriculum design of your particular school. However, most schools offer the following courses in one form or another. We have grouped them into (1) the "preclinical years," or basic science courses covering material tested on Step 1 of the United States Medical Licensing Examination (USMLE); (2) the "clinical years," or courses (clerkships) covering material tested on Step 2 of the USMLE; and (3) the "first postgraduate year," (PGY-1), a brief description covering the material tested on Step 3 of the USMLE. In addition to the courses listed below, most medical schools offer, either as separate courses or within other courses, instruction in: AIDS, alcohol and substance abuse, computer applications in medicine, medical cost containment, death and dying, geriatrics, medical ethics, nutrition, occupational medicine, the physician-patient relationship, preventive medicine, and transfusion medicine. For specific information about the curriculum of each of the 126 medical schools of the United States and Canada, see the Curriculum Directory published each year by the Association of American Medical Colleges (AAMC):

AAMC Curriculum Directory, Association of American Medical Colleges, 2450 N. Street, NW, Washington, DC 20037-1126.

The preclinical years – The first two years of most (traditional) medical curricula include the courses that are listed in this section. The number of hours of class-time shown for each subject are averages from the AAMC. Actual course time varies widely from school to school.

The courses are listed in the order in which they are usually presented during the first two years. Thus, at most schools, students begin their medical education with anatomy, biochemistry, and physiology. From these subjects, which essentially present the "normal" structure and function of the human body, the curriculum proceeds to the basis of disease and treatment. The bulk of the material you study during the preclinical years is basic medical science, the scientific foundation, or basis for medicine.

A very general description of the usual content for each course follows. A detailed content outline for USMLE Step 1 covering all of the basic sciences taught in the first two years of medical school is published each year and can be obtained by writing for the following booklet:

> *USMLE Step 1 General Instructions, Content Outline, and Sample Items*, Philadelphia, The Federation of State Medical Boards of the United States, Inc. and the National Board of Medical Examiners, 1992.

Remember that the courses in your school may rearrange specific topics under different course names or order. In general, the following is an accurate listing of the content of the modern preclinical curriculum. Use this content listing to help organize your study materials as you work your way through your own curriculum. By always thinking in an integrative, systems approach to the basic sciences, you will better understand the basis of medicine.

Gross Anatomy – approximately 180 hours – Gross Anatomy is often the first course taught in medical school. In this course, by far the largest amount of time is spent in the laboratory where students dissect a human cadaver. Emphasis is placed on learning and remembering the names of structures and their anatomical relationships. Often, Gross Anatomy is taught in conjunction with a course in Embryology: there you learn about the origin of the human structure as it develops from fertilized ovum to fetus to neonate to adult form. The Gross Anatomy course is usually organized into sections related to an area of the body and includes thorax, abdomen, pelvis, extremities and back, and head and neck.

While the study of anatomy may seem tedious and not particularly relevant, remember that you must know the structure of the cardiovascular system, for example, before you can study the normal functioning of that system and then the various abnormal processes you will treat as a physician (for example, hypertension). Moreover, those of you who become surgeons, or who perform minor surgery, must know, in great detail and accuracy, the anatomy of the region of the body where you are working. Obviously, surgeons will learn anatomy again at a later time, but your first course in Gross Anatomy sets the stage for much of what you will study and do in the remainder of your medical education.

Neuroanatomy – approximately 80 hours – While the AAMC lists Neuroanatomy as a separate course, many medical schools present this subject as a part of a larger integrated course in Neuroscience that also includes neurophysiology, neuropathology and, sometimes, neuropharmacology. Neuroscience courses often cover such major topics as brain gross anatomy, development of the nervous system, structure and function of the neuron, structure and function of the synapse, the chemistry and function of the neurotransmitters, structure of the spinal cord and its function, the structure and function of the autonomic nervous system, the structure and function of the brainstem and the cranial nerves, sensory systems, forebrain anatomy, motor systems, and a catchall category usually called something like "higher functions of the brain." Neuroanatomy, and, indeed, all of Neuroscience, is required as a foundation for much of what you will do as a doctor. The nervous system controls all the other systems of the body. If you, as a physician, can understand and control the nervous system, you can effectively intervene in such widely diverse problems as mental disease, hypertension, pain, stroke, and fever.

Microanatomy – approximately 100 hours – Microanatomy includes the material taught in Histology and Cell Biology courses in most medical schools. In Histology, the emphasis is on the structure of tissues and how to differentiate one from another. Usually most of your time is spent in the laboratory using a microscope to observe prepared slides of the various tissues. Learning tissue structure and developing an ability to recognize specific tissues is important preparation for later discussions of function in Physiology and recognition of disease states in Pathology. Histology courses are usually divided into units that include the study of epithelium, connective tissue, bone and cartilage, muscle, the nervous system (if not taught in a Neuroscience course), the cardiovascular system including blood and bone marrow, the lymphoid system and cellular immunology, the respiratory system, the integumentary system, the gastrointestinal tract and glands, the endocrine system, the male and female reproductive systems, the urinary system, and the eye and ear. Cell Biology courses (or these topics within Histology courses) look at the structure and function of cellular membranes, cytoplasm and cytoplasmic structures, and the nucleus. The broad field of molecular biology is often introduced with these courses. In this subject, students learn about the structure and functioning of DNA and RNA, the mediators of genetic information.

Biochemistry – approximately 120 hours – Biochemistry is the study of the nature and function of the underlying chemical structure of the cell. Students entering medical school are generally required to have studied both General and Organic Chemistry. You may have taken at least one Biochemistry course or indeed, have majored in biochemistry. Medical schools vary widely in the structure and content of their biochemistry courses. Some are able to place students in introductory or advanced sections, depending upon their particular background. Whatever the level of teaching, most biochemistry courses present the structures and functions of amino acids, proteins, enzymes, nucleic acids, carbohydrates, lipids, vitamins, and hormones. Biochemistry courses usually also include discussions of cell and molecular biology, including membranes, cell structure, and genetic processes. General metabolism and even nutrition may be presented in Biochemistry. It should be obvious that your Biochemistry course contains the chemical basis for essentially everything you will need to understand throughout medicine. You will put your biochemistry knowledge to work in your Physiology course and it will also be important in Microbiology, Pharmacology, etc.

Physiology – approximately 140 hours – Physiology is the study of function. As such, it represents the key to your understanding of medicine. If you do not understand how the body functions normally, you will never be able to understand abnormal function and treatment. Your Physiology course will probably contain only a few laboratory sessions, although traditionally this was a laboratory science. Modern Physiology courses present material mostly in lecture or small group format, with many correlations to clinical material and patient problems. In Anatomy you are asked to learn the details of structure, in Physiology that knowledge will be assumed and you must consider the details of the functioning of structure. Merely memorizing details will not be enough for this course; you must also understand concepts and be able to solve problems. The content of Physiology is usually divided into units of metabolism and endocrinology, the cardiovascular system, the respiratory system, renal physiology and acid-base metabolism, the gastrointestinal system, cellular physiology, and neurophysiology. At many medical schools, the last two topics are taught in other courses (Histology/Cell Biology, Biochemistry, or Neuroscience, for example).

Microbiology – approximately 120 hours – Microbiology is the study of microorganisms, especially those that cause disease in humans. Topics covered include virology, bacteriology, rickettsiae, chlamydiae, mycoplasmas, mycology, and parasitology. Microbiology courses require you to learn taxonomy, anatomy, physiology, and often, pharmacology of microorganisms. Basic immunology may be taught within the Microbiology course, although the current trend in medical education seems to be to present a separate Immunology course for this important and rapidly growing field of medical science.

Immunology – approximately 80 hours – Immunology is the study of the immune system of humans. Many of the topics of this course may be presented within the Biochemistry and Microbiology courses. However, over the last several years there has been a rapid growth in the understanding of the details of immunology and their importance in understanding disease and medicine. Most medical schools now offer a separate course in this important subject.

Genetics – approximately 35 hours – In many medical schools, Genetics is incorporated within other courses, but the recent trend has been to offer a separate course. This course often begins with the molecular basis of genetics (cell biology) and proceeds through simple Mendelian inheritance, chromosomal inheritance, population genetics, and polygenic inheritance. Clinical genetics and reproductive genetics are usually taught using representative patient cases. Students are expected to learn about the many inherited diseases of humans during this course. Ethical issues and genetic counseling are often discussed.

Pathology – approximately 160 hours – Pathology includes both the "anatomy" and the "physiology" of disease. This course (or series of courses) usually begins with topics in general pathology, which include mechanisms of disease, healing, inflammation, etc. The anatomical portion of pathology is taught at both the gross and the histological level. Diseases and their effects on tissues and organs usually are studied in a system-by-system manner. Thus, Pathology courses generally contain sections on hematology; the cardiovascular, respiratory, gastrointestinal, endocrine, genitourinary, nervous, and musculoskeletal systems; the skin; and the breast. Pathology is the first course where you will study diseases and disease mechanisms in both a specific and a comprehensive manner. This important course provides the basics so you can understand the diagnosis, treatment, and management of patients with disease.

Pharmacology – approximately 110 hours – Pharmacology deals with the effects of drugs on both normal physiology and the altered physiology of disease states. In this course you learn the general principles of drug administration, transport, storage, action, degradation, and excretion. You also learn about toxic substances, how they affect the body, are metabolized and excreted, and how to treat patients suffering from their effects. Generally, Pharmacology courses are presented in a system-by-system order, with the classes of drugs grouped together based on their chemistry, action, or target. For each drug, you need to know something about its chemical structure, route of administration, dosage, transport, target, duration of activity, and route of elimination. You also study the side effects of each drug and any effects of their interactions with other drugs. All in all, this course challenges your memory and good study habits because it includes so many details about a large number of different drugs as well as many concepts and principles relating drug actions and physiology.

Epidemiology – approximately 60 hours – Epidemiology is the study of the distribution and occurrence of diseases. Within this course you learn how diseases spread through populations, demographic characteristics, geographic distributions, modes of disease transmission, risk factors for disease, and prevention of disease. While studying epidemiology, you also learn the details of biostatistics, the concepts of measurement in medicine, as well as study design, and the interpretation of medical literature. These important topics permit you to read articles about clinical trials of drugs and other treatments and correctly interpret the results of the studies. In many medical schools, the study of epidemiology is found within a more general course on community medicine.

Behavioral Science – approximately 60 hours – Most medical schools offer study in behavioral science or medical psychology either as a separate course or within other courses. The content of behavioral science usually includes the biological correlates of behavior, behavioral genetics, personality, learning and behavioral change, life-span development, communication and interaction, group processes, family and community, sociocultural patterns of behavior, behavioral risk factors and disease, health care systems, and behavioral statistics and design. Wherever it is taught in your school, it is important, not only for the insight it gives you but also because behavioral science topics represent a significant portion of USMLE Step 1.

Summary of the preclinical years – While you generally study the basic sciences in a course-by-course manner, keep in mind that all of the material is interrelated. You will be tested in a more or less integrative manner on Step 1 of the USMLE and you should prepare for this exam from the very beginning. For more extensive information about how to study and review specifically for Step 1 see:

> Thornborough, J. R., Schmidt, H. J., *How to Prepare for the Step 1 Medical Exam*, 2nd ed., New York, NY, McGraw-Hill, 1993.

The clinical years – The second two years of medical school are usually occupied with clinical clerkships and electives. For the most part, the clerkships are scheduled in the third year. During the bulk of the fourth year, students take electives in areas of special interest and visit schools and hospitals where they may wish to do their residency. The fourth year is also used for interviewing at residency programs in preparation for the residency match process that occurs in February.

For each course a very general description of the usual content is presented below. A much more detailed content outline for USMLE Step 2, which covers all of the clinical sciences taught in the second two years of medical school, is published each year in the following booklet:

> *USMLE Step 2 General Instructions, Content Outline, and Sample Items*, Philadelphia, The Federation of State Medical Boards of the United States, Inc. and the National Board of Medical Examiners.

Family/Community Medicine – approximately five to six weeks – Clinical rotations in family medicine and/or community medicine are offered by most medical schools. There is a great amount of variation in what is presented within this subject area, but it usually includes time spent in outpatient clinics and/or private physicians' offices. Topics include determinants of health care policy, health care financing, health promotion, health surveys, disease reporting mechanisms, public health issues, environmental health, occupational health, legal and ethical issues, etc. Some schools have special programs in family medicine.

Physical Diagnosis – four to eight weeks – Sir William Osler wrote, ". . . teach the eye to see, the finger to feel, and the ear to hear." This succinctly states the goal of the course in Physical Diagnosis. You learn to take a patient's medical history and to carefully inspect, palpate, percuss, and listen to their body. You study the general appearance of both normal and disease states of the head, eyes, ears, nose, throat; the cardiovascular system, thorax, abdomen; the musculoskeletal system; the reproductive system; the skin; and the nervous system. Often this course is presented within the first two years of medicine (the preclinical years). Physical Diagnosis can be called "Introduction to the Patient," "Introduction to Clinical Medicine," "Clinical Assessment," etc.

Medicine – approximately twelve weeks – Medicine is usually one of the longest clerkships in medical school and certainly is the foundation for much of medical practice. You learn to admit and work up the history of patients with problems in a variety of areas, including: allergy, immunology, infectious diseases, rheumatology, pulmonary disease, cardiology, endocrinology and metabolic disease, gastroenterology, nephrology, oncology and hematology, neurology, and dermatology. You work with a preceptor who is a resident in medicine. Teaching in the medicine clerkship, as in most of the clinical courses, is mostly done by demonstration from your preceptor followed by supervised practice on your part.

Neurology – approximately four weeks – During your neurology clerkship, you learn to perform a neurologic examination and to perform and interpret various diagnostic tests. All physicians, regardless of their speciality, use these techniques and skills when examining a patient. They represent an important view of what is going on in a person's body since the nervous system is involved in the control and operation of all of the other systems. Most neurology rotations include a study of cerebrovascular disease, epilepsy and seizures, headache and facial pain, traumatic and occupational injuries, infections of the nervous system, neoplasms of the nervous system, nutritional and metabolic disorders of the nervous system, degenerative disorders, demyelinating disorders, developmental and hereditary disorders, neuromuscular disorders, toxic injuries, eye disease and visual disturbances, disturbances of hearing, balance, smell, and taste, spinal cord and root disease, peripheral neuropathy, and the management of neurological disorders.

Obstetrics and Gynecology – approximately seven weeks – During your Ob/Gyn clerkship you learn to deliver babies and experience the wonderful satisfaction and thrill of actually doing so. This clerkship also covers such topics as the anatomy, genetics, and embryology of the developing fetus, ultrasound and congenital anomalies, puberty, menstruation, menopause, sexuality, conception, diagnostic procedures, contraception, abortion, and sterilization. You study the normal fetus, placenta, newborn, normal pregnancy, labor, delivery, and puerperium, spontaneous abortion, ectopic pregnancies, trophoblastic disease, medical, surgical, and obstetric complications of pregnancy, diagnosis and management of disorders of labor, delivery, and puerperium, menstrual and endocrine disorders, pelvic relaxation, gynecological infections, endometriosis and infertility, and the treatment of benign and malignant neoplasms.

Pediatrics – approximately eight weeks – Pediatrics encompasses the care of children ranging in age from neonates through adolescents. It includes care for both well children and ill children. Topics usually covered include well care and general pediatrics; care for the newborn infant; the cardiovascular, respiratory, gastrointestinal, urinary, and neuromuscular systems; infectious diseases and immunology; hematologic and neoplastic diseases; endocrine, and genetic disorders; and care of the adolescent.

Psychiatry – approximately six to seven weeks – Psychiatry includes the use of both psychotherapy and psychopharmacology. During your psychiatry clerkship you learn the details and techniques for evaluation, assessment, and diagnosis of psychiatric patients. You also study human behavior; theories of personality and development; organic mental disorders; schizophrenia, delusional, and other psychotic disorders; mood disorders; anxiety; somatoform and dissociative disorders; personality disorders; human sexuality; alcoholism and substance abuse; and law and ethics in Psychiatry.

Radiology – approximately two to three weeks – Radiology is taught as a separate course during the clinical years in only a few medical schools. In Radiology, you learn to recognize structures in X-ray images, MRIs, CAT scans, etc. Radiology courses also offer instruction in the therapeutic use of various forms of radiation. If your school does not offer a separate Radiology course, you learn about these topics in such courses as Anatomy, Pathology,

Medicine, etc. Also, you may be able to take an elective in Radiology during your fourth year.

Surgery – approximately twelve weeks – Surgery, like Medicine, is usually a major component of your clinical training. During your surgery rotation, you spend time observing and assisting with surgical procedures on patients. Thus, you learn to scrub, to name various surgical instruments and their functions, to tie surgical knots, etc. Topics studied usually include pre- and postoperative care, critical care, anesthesiology, blood gases, respiratory care, wounds, infections, and burns of the skin, plastic surgery, trauma and shock, transplantation, immunology, oncology, endocrine problems, breast, the gastrointestinal tract, liver and pancreas, cardiothoracic problems, and peripheral vascular problems.

Specialties – These are usually short clerkships through which students rotate in the third or fourth year of medical school. Some medical schools offer them in a block while others present them as more complete individual courses. The specialties, as we define them, include Anesthesiology, Urology, Orthopedics, Neurosurgery, and Otolaryngology.

First postgraduate year – During the first postgraduate year (internship), most new graduate MDs are occupied with patient care duties within their residency. Under the supervision of more senior residents and attending physicians, you learn to care for patients. By the end of the year, you should have acquired sufficient knowledge and skill to practice without the need for supervision. This year will prepare you to pass Step 3 of the USMLE and thus complete the requirements to become a licensed physician and be permitted by law to practice medicine without the need for direct supervision.

A detailed content outline for USMLE Step 3, which lists all of the skills, techniques, diseases, and patient management approaches you must learn during your first postgraduate year (as well as in medical school), is published each year in the following booklet:

USMLE Step 3 General Instructions, Content Outline, and Sample Items, Philadelphia, The Federation of State Medical Boards of the United States, Inc. and the National Board of Medical Examiners.

Chapter 4

Financing Your Medical Education

Introduction – In addition to all the time and effort required by medical school, you must also be concerned about the expense of your education. Not only is tuition high, but activity fees, housing costs, medical instruments, books, application fees, testing fees, and travel expenses all add up to a significant amount. By now, most of you will have made financial arrangements for your first year through your school's financial aid office. The purpose of this chapter is to help you plan for the remaining years of your medical education and to give you some ideas for additional financing. Most important, spend some time with a person in your school's financial aid office. These people are trained to help you with money matters and are knowledgeable about financial programs available to medical students.

Making a budget – In money matters, most surprises are bad news. Winning the lottery or the Publishers' Clearing House Sweepstakes would be nice but the chances of this happening are rather slim. The kinds of surprises you are more likely to encounter include an unexpected bill for health insurance, $500 for required books, major expenses for medical instruments needed in Physical Diagnosis, $700 airfare to visit a residency program for an interview, etc. Most "surprise" expenses need not be a surprise, however, since this chapter will help you estimate most of them and create a reasonably accurate budget. Make out your budget immediately and get your money matters in order. If you estimate that you will not have enough money for your expenses, make an appointment with your school's financial aid officer to go over your budget and discuss loan possibilities, etc. Be sure to update and revise your budget periodically. Income and expenses may change and your budget should reflect these fluctuations. Plan carefully so you won't be unpleasantly surprised, you have more important things to think about than money problems.

Estimating your income – As a full-time medical student, you probably will not be able to work much to generate a significant income. You will have to rely on savings, help from your family, scholarships, and loans. The issue is, even with all of these sources of income, will you have enough money? To answer this question, first add up all of the income you know you can count on for the next four years. Use the budget table for income estimation on the following page. Be as accurate as possible and do not enter amounts that you "think" you may have. Enter only the money you know you can count on. It is important to differentiate between loans from family and friends and gifts that you will not have to repay. Enter the amounts you will receive each year and also a four-year total for each category. Finally, add the categories to obtain an overall four-year total of income. You may wish to decrease this total by 10% to be on the safe side.

NOTE: If there are significant differences in the amount of income you will receive in different years, you may wish to calculate an income total for each of the four years. Your expenses will vary somewhat but large items such as tuition, housing, and food will remain relatively constant. If you expect to have a very small income in a particular year, even though your four-year total is sufficient, then you must plan ahead to avoid a "cash flow" problem.

Estimating your expenses – On the following budget pages, we have divided the expenses into two major categories: (1) those related to medical school; and (2) those required for general living expenses. When estimating your expenses be as accurate as possible. In some cases you will have exact figures and in others you must guess. If you guess, err on the high side. It is better to find something costs less than what you planned, rather than the opposite. Your medical school's financial aid office can help you estimate the cost of books, supplies, and instruments. Upper class students can also be a source of information. Get all the help you can in completing your budget; an accurate budget will save you headaches later on.

Medical school expenses – Enter figures on a monthly basis when appropriate. Tuition is the largest item. Ask your financial aid office for information on estimated increases. Most medical schools charge a fixed fee for student activities, breakage deposits, malpractice insurance, etc. Enter estimates for books, instruments, and supplies. During your second year, you must pay for the USMLE Step 1 examination and during your fourth year, Step 2. In the fourth year, you also will apply for residency programs and will have to travel for interviews. Costs of travel will depend somewhat on your plans. For example, if you are going to medical school in California and plan to do your residency on the east coast, then you must plan for some serious travel expenses.

NOTE: Be sure to use the time line in Chapter 2 when making out your budget. Special expenses related to examinations, interviews, etc., can be located in time and will help with your financial planning.

BUDGET

Income

Source	Amount per Year	4-Year Total
Family gift(s)		
–	_____	_____
–	_____	_____
–	_____	_____
Family loan(s)		
–	_____	_____
–	_____	_____
–	_____	_____
Savings		
–	_____	_____
–	_____	_____
Job(s)		
–	_____	_____
–	_____	_____
–	_____	_____
Loan(s)		
–	_____	_____
–	_____	_____
–	_____	_____
–	_____	_____
–	_____	_____
Scholarship(s)		
–	_____	_____
–	_____	_____
–	_____	_____
–	_____	_____

4-YearTotal: [_____]

BUDGET

Expenses

Category	Monthly	Yearly
MEDICAL SCHOOL		
Tuition		
–	_____	_____
Activity Fee		
–	_____	_____
Books		
–	_____	_____
Instruments		
–	_____	_____
Supplies		
–	_____	_____
Application Fees		
–	_____	_____
Travel		
–	_____	_____
LIVING		
Housing		
–	_____	_____
Telephone		
–	_____	_____
Electricity		
–	_____	_____
Water/Sewer		
–	_____	_____
Heat		
–	_____	_____
Food		
–	_____	_____

BUDGET

Expenses

Category	Monthly	Yearly
Entertainment		
–	_____	_____
Clothing		
–	_____	_____
Automobile		
–	_____	_____
Gasoline		
–	_____	_____
Insurance		
auto–	_____	_____
life–	_____	_____
health–	_____	_____
property–	_____	_____
other–	_____	_____
Loan Repayment		
–	_____	_____
Credit Card(s)		
–	_____	_____
Presents		
–	_____	_____
Travel		
–	_____	_____
Other		
–	_____	_____
–		

Yearly Total: [＿＿＿＿＿＿]

4-Year Total: [＿＿＿＿＿＿]

General living expenses – This general category of expenses contains everything concerning your life maintenance. As before, you should try to enter figures on a monthly basis. Not all categories will necessarily apply to you and you may think of some special ones that we have not included. The point of this is to list every expense you will have over the next four years.

Calculate your balance – When you have finished entering expense items, add up the columns and enter the yearly and the four-year total. It is probably wise to increase your total expenses by 10% to cover items you may have forgotten as well as possible inflationary increases. You may wish to calculate a separate total for each year if you find that some years are more expensive that others. Compare your four-year expense total to your four-year income total. If income is larger, congratulations. If income is smaller, then you should immediately go to your school's financial aid office to review your budget and find a solution to your shortfall.

A final word about your budget – Your three largest expenses will be tuition, housing, and food and the amounts of these are relatively fixed. If you look for places in your budget to enact savings, these items can only be adjusted minimally. You may be able to find cheaper housing, but don't forget the benefits of living in medical school housing with your colleagues. Also, you can't really eat less, although you can eat somewhat more cheaply. All in all, your budget will be relatively inflexible and you should plan now for sufficient funds to cover your expenses. If you do plan carefully, money will be one less worry you will have while you are studying medicine.

Loans and scholarships – The best source of information about available loans and scholarships is your medical school's financial aid office. However, the following list presents several sources that may be of interest to you:

Medloans Residency Relocation and Internship Interview Travel Expense Loan gives small loans (up to $7,000) to fourth-year medical students for travel expenses to visit and interview at various residency programs and for relocation to your residency.

Your medical school probably has a private source of funds for scholarships and loans. You should explore this possibility with your school's financial aid advisor.

Native Americans are eligible for financial aid from the United States Department of the Interior, Bureau of Indian Affairs, New York Liaison Office, Federal Building, Room 523, 100 South Clinton Street, Syracuse, New York 13202. Try contacting them for information.

Most states have financial assistance programs of one sort or another for residents who are medical students. You should contact your state's education department or your medical school's financial aid office for information.

State, and county, medical societies often offer financial assistance to medical students. Contact them for information.

For fourth-year medical students, the National Health Service Corporation Loan Repayment Program will pay up to $35,000 a year toward your medical education loans if you agree to a two-year, full-time practice at an NHSC or Indian Health Service site. Contact: Division of Health Services Scholarships, Rm. 7-16, Parklawn Building, 5600 Fishers Lane, Rockville, MD 20857, Telephone: (301) 443-1650.

The Armed Forces Health Professions Scholarship Programs offer tuition, fees, and a stipend to medical students that obligates them to active duty in one of the services. Write to the service of your choice for information and an application:

Department of the Army, Office of the Surgeon General, DASG-PTP, Washington, DC 20314.

Department of the Navy, Bureau of Medicine and Surgery, Attn.: Code 3174, Washington, DC 20372.

Department of the Air Force, HQ ATC/RSOS, Randolph Air Force Base, Texas 78148.

You may obtain information about the Veterans Administration Health Professions Scholarship Program from: Affiliated Education Programs Service, Office of Academic Affairs, Department of Medicine and Surgery, Veterans Administration, 810 Vermont Avenue, N.W., Washington, DC 20420.

Health Professions Scholarships for Students of Exceptional Financial Need and Program of Financial Assistance for Disadvantaged Health Professions Students are federal programs administered by medical schools. Ask your financial aid office.

Charities, foundations, service and religious organizations, labor unions, and philanthropic groups are possible sources of financial aid. Ask those in your community for information and get help from your school's financial aid office.

Jewish Foundation for Education of Women, 330 West 58 Street, New York, NY 10019, Telephone: (212) 265-2565 has grants and loans for female students according to financial need.

National Medical Fellowships, 254 West 31 Street, New York, NY 10019, Telephone: (212) 714-0933 offers grants to minority medical students.

Grants for minority medical students are offered by the Women's Auxiliary to the National Medical Association, 150 West End Ave., New York, NY 10023.

Grants for women medical students are available from the Alpha Epsilon Iota Scholarship Fund, Ann Arbor Trust Company, P.O. Box 12, Ann Arbor, MI 48107.

Fourth-year female medical students should apply in the fall of their third year for grants from the American Association of University Women, Education Foundation, 2401 Virginia Avenue, N.W., Washington, DC 20037.

Small scholarships based on academics and need are offered by the American Educational Services, Scholarship Program Director, 419 Lentz Court, Lansing, MI 48917.

Japanese Medical Society of America, One Henry St., Englewood Cliffs, NJ 07632 offers scholarships based on need.

Doctors Care International Foundation offers scholarships based on financial need. Contact: Grants Department, P.O. Box 1111, Houston, Texas 77251-1111.

Stephen Bufton Memorial Educational Fund, American Business Women's Association, 9100 Ward Parkway, Kansas City, MO 64114 has small scholarships for women students.

Students of Hispanic background may contact the National Hispanic Scholarship Fund, P.O. Box 728, Novato, CA 94948.

National Italian American Foundation, 666 11th St., N.W., Suite 800, Washington, DC 20001, Telephone: (202) 638-0220.

The financial aid office of your medical school can give you information about National Direct (Perkins) Student Loans. These are based upon need and have a maximum of $18,000.

You should contact the Education Department of your state of residence as well as local lending institutions for information about loan programs appropriate for medical students.

The federal Health Education Assistance (HEAL) Loan Program offers loans up to $20,000 a year for your four years of medical school. See your school's financial aid office for details.

The Association of American Medical Colleges provides the MEDLOANS Program, which permits you to borrow through the Stafford Guaranteed Student Loan (GSL), Supplemental Loans for Students (SLS), and the Alternative Loan Program (ALP). These loan programs provide as much as $30,000 per year for your four years of medical school. Ask your financial aid office for information about all of the options.

The Family Ed loan program from the Student Loan Marketing Association (SALLIE MAE) offers medical students yearly loans of up to $10,000 per year for four years. These are regular consumer loans requiring good credit and a substantial income. You will probably have to use a co-borrower for this loan. See your medical school's financial aid office.

National Association of Residents and Interns has loans of $5,000 or $10,000 if you have signed a residency contract: 292 Madison Avenue, New York, NY 10017.

American Medical Student Association offers loans up to $5,000 if you have signed a residency contract: P.O. Box 131, 14650 Lee Rd., Chantilly, VA 22021, (800) 336-0158.

Medical Education Life Fund, Inc. offers loans to junior and senior students: Box 5347, Charlottesville, VA 22903.

The United States Medical Advisory Association has a program for senior students offering loans up to $15,000: P.O. Box 200, 110 S. Poplar Street, Wilmington, DE 19801, Telephone: (800) 223-7076.

Max Thorek Student Loan Fund, International College of Surgeons, 1516 Lake Shore Drive, Chicago, IL 60610.

Albert Strickler Memorial Fund, 1006 LaFayette Building, Philadelphia, PA 19106.

Hattie M. Strong Foundation, Att: Director of Loans, 1625 Eye Street, N.W., Suite 409, Washington, DC 20006.

Medical Student's Aid Society, Phi Lambda Kappa Medical Society, Rm. 1400, 1015 Chestnut St., Philadelphia, PA 19107.

Mediclinics Educational Fund, 2000 Midwest Plaza Building, Minneapolis, MN 55402.

Presbyterian Church Higher Education Loan Fund, 34 Ponce de Leon Avenue, N.W., Atlanta, GA 30308.

United Methodist Student Loan Fund, P.O. Box 871, Nashville, TN 37202.

Loan repayment – You will probably find it necessary to borrow money throughout your four years of medical school. The sources of these loans may include

• family and friends who loan you money, with or without interest that you must pay back.

• regular commercial loans with interest that must be paid on a schedule that begins when you receive the money.

• special loans that require you to pay interest from the beginning, but allow you to defer payments on principal until you earn an income.

• special loans that permit you to defer payment of both interest and principal until you have finished school.

Calculating your monthly or quarterly payments for combinations of these loan types can be a formidable task. However, you must at least estimate what your payments will be so that you can budget your money accurately when you begin your residency. For loans requiring you to pay principal and/or interest during medical school, you must enter your monthly payments into the budget calculations described earlier in this chapter. To calculate payments for deferred loans over the 10 years after you graduate, use the conversion factors in the following table. See the sample calculation that illustrates how to find a single monthly payment for three loans, each with a different principal amount and interest rate.

**TABLE OF CONVERSION RATES
FOR A 10-YEAR
REPAYMENT SCHEDULE**

Interest Rate	Conversion Rate
3%	0.009656
4%	0.010125
5%	0.010607
7%	0.011611
8%	0.012133
9%	0.012668
12%	0.014347
14%	0.015527
16%	0.016751
18%	0.018018

A sample repayment schedule – If you borrow $10,000 at 5% interest, $7,000 at 12% interest, and $15,000 at 14% interest, your repayment of the loans over a 10-year period would be calculated as follows:

5% monthly repayment: $10,000 x 0.010607 = $106.07
12% monthly repayment: $7,000 x 0.014347 = $100.43
14% monthly repayment: $15,000 x 0.015527 = $232.91

Total Estimated Monthly Repayment: **$439.41**

Chapter 5

Basic Supplies for Your Study Desk

Introduction – Be sure you have a personal study area where you can keep your books, notes, etc. Wherever you live (dormitory, apartment, with spouse or family), it is important to define a private work area where you know everything you need is available and where it will always be quiet and conducive to serious studying. Below is a list of some of the general necessities for your "office."

White, 8½" × 11" ruled pads – Make your notes from classes on these as well as notes and summaries you make when you study. Buy the pads with three holes punched or get a punch of your own and save all of your notes in loose-leaf binders. With your notes loose, you can reorganize them as your needs for the information change. For example, you may keep your Physiology notes in a binder organized as the course is organized, system by system. This way you can easily integrate your notes with handouts, syllabus material and transcripts from the course. Later, when you take Pharmacology, you may want to incorporate your Physiology notes into your Pharmacology binders. This way you can review the Physiology as you study the effects of drugs on systems. Finally, you may decide to merge both Physiology and Pharmacology notes into your materials for Medicine, allowing for another review of these subjects as you study disease and treatment.

Pencils – Have a supply of several well-sharpened pencils with erasers handy for calculations, temporary study notes, thoughts, ideas, and doodles. Get yourself a pencil sharpener (any will do, from a cheap, hand-operated model to an expensive electric sharpener). As you study, pause now and then to jot down ideas, make a table, or graph data. Try rearranging the information to see it from a different perspective. These are all "active learning" devices that will help you understand and remember material (see Chapter 10 for specific information about how to study most efficiently). Most of these penciled jottings can be thrown away at the end of each study session, but you may want to copy over in ink and save some of your more useful summaries. These will be very important later on when you are reviewing for an exam. Finally, you will need No. 2 pencils for computer-graded exams.

Ball point pens (black, blue, red, green, etc.) – Do most of your basic note keeping in black ink and use the other colors for items you wish to emphasize or for complex drawings.

Highlighter – Use highlighters carefully. It's good to highlight important points in your textbooks and notes, but if you find yourself coloring almost the whole page, stop. It means the textbook is densely packed with information and you are failing to select appropriate material for highlighting. Try taking notes and reorganizing the information in a different form so that relationships are easier for you to remember. Whatever you do, avoid creating "jaundiced" or "psychedelic" textbooks (see Chapter 10).

Dictionary – It should be obvious that a good dictionary of the English language is necessary for any intellectual pursuit, including the study of medicine. Check your spelling for every word you aren't sure of – even in your own notes. In this way, you constantly improve your spelling and vocabulary. If you must write a lot of reports and papers, you may also wish to have a thesaurus.

Webster's Ninth New Collegiate Dictionary, Springfield, IL, Merriam-Webster, Inc., 1991.

Webster's College Dictionary and College Thesaurus, New York, NY, Random House, 1992.

Chapman, R.L., Ed., *Roget's International Thesaurus*, 5th ed., New York, NY, Harper Collins, 1992.

Medical dictionary – This is your most basic and necessary reference. Buy one (there are several good ones) your first time in the bookstore and keep it handy. Do not "read through" unknown words – look them up.

Hensyl, W.R., ed., *Stedman's Medical Dictionary*, 25th ed., Baltimore, Md., Williams & Wilkins, 1990.

Dorland's Illustrated Medical Dictionary, 27th ed., Orlando, Fla., W.B. Saunders Company, 1993.

Tape recorder – Portable cassette tape recorders are relatively inexpensive and you should find room in your supplies budget for one. You may wish to record certain lectures, etc., but be careful. Remember, it takes just as long to listen to a recording of an hour lecture as it did to sit in the lecture with your tape recorder. Always take notes. If you find your note-taking skills inadequate, you may want to record lectures so that you can fill in bare spots later. You won't need to listen to the entire recording, just the parts where your notes are weak. Also, students at many medical schools operate a note-taking service whereby all classes are recorded and written transcripts are available within a few days. However, even if you have a note-taking service, take your own notes. Later, use the transcripts to supplement your own active, writing-down of information while in class. (See Chapter 8 for how to use your student transcript service effectively.)

One valuable use of a tape recorder is to make your own review tapes. Construct "lectures" for yourself by organizing the material from class notes, textbook readings, etc., and then give your lecture to your tape recorder. Later, when you are commuting or traveling, listen to yourself explain material you need to review. Does it still make sense? Were you correct when you made the tape? Has subsequent study changed your view of the material? Making your own review tapes forces you to think about and organize information. This is a form of active learning. Hearing yourself say on tape things you once thought about and organized is a powerful stimulus for recall. Try it, we think you will find this form of studying very helpful.

The New England Journal of Medicine – This weekly journal of general medicine published since 1812 contains original research articles, reviews, presentations of images in clinical medicine, case records, letters, editorials, and book reviews. Read it every week. You may not understand everything you read but you will find it interesting and it adds to your general fund of medical knowledge. If you find an article that interests you but you don't understand, use your medical dictionary for unknown terms and read *Harrison's* (see below) for background information.

Reading journals should become a lifelong endeavor that will help to keep you current with the many, rapidly occurring changes in medicine. To obtain a subscription to *The New England Journal of Medicine,* write:

The New England Journal of Medicine
P.O. Box 9150
Waltham, MA 02254-9150
or Telephone: 1-800-THE NEJM

Harrison's Principles of Internal Medicine – Buy this classic book of medicine your first year and make it a practice to read about every disease, patient, treatment, or condition that may be discussed, used as an example, or just mentioned in your classes. You don't need to take notes or attempt to learn the details – that will come later – but read it for general background information. This practice will help you remember and generally add to your fund of knowledge. Furthermore, this practice can help you maintain interest by orienting "irrelevant" basic sciences in clinical facts. Below is the complete reference for this important book:

> Wilson, J. D. et al., *Harrison's Principles of Internal Medicine*, 12th Ed., New York, N.Y., McGraw-Hill, 1991.

Miscellaneous – You will need paper clips, fasteners, erasers, scissors, a ruler, a multi-function calculator, a good reading lamp, 3-ring loose-leaf binders for keeping your notes, file folders, 3" × 5" file cards, a stapler, scotch tape, a book shelf, bookends, and a file cabinet (inexpensive, plastic "milk crates" substitute quite nicely).

Interpreting the Medical Literature – This is a brief, easy-to-read book that should be on your desk when you are studying or reading journals. It contains information on how to evaluate the design and execution of clinical studies, how to critically analyze and interpret data, and a good introduction to basic statistics. You will find this book invaluable later on when you take epidemiology:

> Gehlbach, S. H., *Interpreting the Medical Literature,* 3rd ed., New York, McGraw-Hill, 1993.

How to Prepare for the Step 1 Medical Exam – This book contains suggestions for undertaking an efficient and effective review of all of your basic science courses. You may want to get this book now and organize your studying in a way that optimizes your review for the Step 1 examination that you must take in a year or so:

> Thornborough, J. R., Schmidt, H. J., *How to Prepare for the Step 1 Medical Exam*, 2nd Ed., New York, N.Y., McGraw-Hill, 1993.

Chapter 6

What to Bring From College

Introduction – While in school, we all tend to study diligently and prepare carefully for a course and its examinations. When the course is over and we have gone on to a new subject, much of what we learned is seldom used again and rather quickly forgotten. However, look upon your college education not only as a hurdle to overcome before entering medical school but also as a provider of information that you will use during your medical studies. In other words, there are many facts, concepts, and skills that you are expected to bring with you when you begin to study medicine.

Below is a list of topics we think are particularly important and which you should understand and review if necessary. Read through the list and make a quick evaluation of how well prepared you are for medical school. Take some time early in your studies to do some remedial reading if necessary.

Algebraic relationships – Simple algebra is used often in medical school to solve many biological problems. You are probably comfortable with these concepts, but if not, it would be wise to undertake a review.

Basic electricity – An understanding of the physical laws governing electricity, the units of potential, current, and resistance is necessary because electrical phenomena are involved in the functioning of all cells, especially nerves and muscles. Review the electricity section of your college Physics courses.

Basic mathematics – Accurately adding, subtracting, multiplying, and dividing are crucial in medical school. Obviously, everyone knows how to add and subtract, so why do we list these skills here? You would be surprised how many medical students are careless in this area. Carefully examine your own record for mathematical accuracy and take steps to improve if necessary.

Chemistry of acids, bases, buffers, and electrolytes – The basic chemical principles describing the behavior of acids, bases, buffers and electrolytes are fundamental to understanding the processes of living organisms. These topics are discussed in several of your courses but you need to recall the basics (see also pH, below).

Diffusion – Diffusion is the net movement of particles (molecules, for example) down their concentration gradient. It is absolutely necessary that you understand this concept as it is used in many physiological processes.

Drawing/reading/interpreting graphs – Teachers, textbooks, scientific journals, and examinations present information visually in graphs. In turn, you will be expected to interpret these and be able to create and draw graphs of your own.

Look through a textbook or journal article for a graph. The specific subject makes no difference. Take a little time to make sure you understand just what it presents. Cover the graph's legend and attempt to write your own. Now read the author's legend and, if necessary, part of the text of the article to see how you did. This exercise will give you valuable practice in interpreting graphs.

A different approach is to find a table of data and attempt to present it (or a part of it) as a graph. This is not only good practice in organizing and presenting data but also an excellent study device to use when preparing for examinations. It is a form of active learning and will help you understand and remember the information. Also, your graph can be saved for future review.

Exponentiation – Related to using logarithms is the ability to express numbers in exponential form. In Biology, numbers are often either very large or very small and thus are presented as exponents (usually of 10). Be sure you can do this operation.

Gas laws – Return to your Physics course and review the gas laws. These are fundamental to the understanding of much of medicine and you will need them early in your studies.

Logarithms – Logarithms (both base 10 and natural) are often used in your medical studies. Take some time to review the subject and make sure you understand the concepts and have some facility in their use. Being prepared to use logs will save you trouble later on.

Metric units of measure – While growing up you probably learned about inches, miles, quarts, pints, pounds, ounces, etc., the units commonly used in the United States. However, scientists and the entire medical community more often use metric units of measure: meters, kilometers, liters, milliliters, kilograms, grams, etc. You will not necessarily have to convert from one system to the other, but you should have the comparisons in mind.

Ohm's law – This law describes the relationship among electrical potential, current, and resistance. A variant of the law describes a similar relationship between pressure, flow, and resistance to flow of fluids. You use Ohm's law during your studies of nerves and nerve conduction and also when you explore how the cardiovascular system maintains a flow of blood, under pressure, to every tissue of the body.

Osmolality – Osmolality and osmotic pressure are concepts that govern the movement of water into and out of cells. This process is vital to the proper functioning of both cells and whole organisms.

pH – You should understand the pH scale for expressing hydrogen ion concentration (acidity or basicity) throughout your medical career. This concept is used immediately in Biochemistry and Physiology, but you continue to need it in all of your medical school courses as well as in treating patients. Take the time early on to review your college Chemistry notes or text and make sure you understand pH.

Probability theory – Probability theory and the rules of chance are necessary to truly understand many of the processes of Biology that you study in medical school. Biostatistics, Epidemiology, and Public Health subjects are included in most medical school curricula and the concepts taught are an extension of probability theory.

Reading quickly and effectively – Probably the most valuable skill you can have (or acquire) is the ability to read rapidly and effectively. In medical school, you must read vast amounts of written material in relatively short periods of time. Your success as a student will depend upon your efficiency in reading rapidly, understanding, and remembering what you have read.

If you feel you are not an efficient reader, you should get help. There are many reading skills classes available as well as self-help books, computer programs, and so forth. The education office at many medical schools may offer help with improving reading skills – find out if your school provides such a service. Do not make the mistake of taking a <u>speed-reading</u> course. While speed-reading may have merit when reading novels or the newspaper, it is <u>not</u> an appropriate method for reading and understanding medical textbooks. (See Chapter 9 for a complete discussion of efficient and effective approaches to reading medical texts.)

Scientific method and rules of evidence – The practice of medicine is the application of scientific knowledge about the normal and pathological functioning of the body to prevent, control, or cure disease and injury. In every instance, the scientific basis for medicine is based on a process of gathering information according to very specific rules: the scientific method. It is beneficial to recall, from time to time, how hypotheses are generated, evidence is gathered, and conclusions supported.

Solutions; molar, equivalent – Learn again the definitions of mole and equivalent. Work out how to make these solutions and what they mean. You need this information over and over again.

Taking notes – No matter how many electronic aids, note-taking services, textbooks, extensive syllabus materials, hand-outs, etc., may be available to you, you should be able to quickly take clear, accurate, and useful notes. And you should actually do it. The act of processing information and writing it in your notes while seeing and hearing a teaching presentation is a valuable, active learning process. Learn to take good notes. See Chapter 9 for how to take good notes and how to develop a system that will <u>not</u> require the, often difficult, integration of several different note sets.

Touch-typing – If you don't already know how, learn to type. You can do so fairly easily and quickly by using one of the many available computer programs that teach touch-typing. Inquire in your library or in the computer center if your school has one. Chances are a typing teaching program is available for your use.

Using a calculator – Having grown up with calculators, most of you are very facile with them. If you are not, learn to use it so well that you can perform calculations without consciously thinking about the specific operations. Remember, you want to solve a problem. You don't want to slow down to figure out how to use the functions of the machine every time you need a number.

Using a library – Most medical schools have an orientation program for entering students that includes a tour of the medical library and information on how to use it. Most libraries are now heavily computerized for location of books, articles, and information, but you must learn how to use the computer's search routines. Be sure to attend the library orientation.

Throughout your career you will need to search for information so learn how to use a library efficiently in your first year in medical school. If yours does not offer special courses for students, be sure to ask for help. With a good medical library behind you, you can access every item of information you ever need to know. When you begin using the medical library, don't hesitate to ask the librarians for help. It is especially important to get their help when you are doing a literature search. These experts are trained in how to properly search the literature and they can provide you with insights that reflect their years of study and experience.

Using a microscope – You probably learned the fundamentals of using a microscope in your college Biology courses. Recall what you learned. Early in most medical curricula, students use microscopes in the Histology course. Later, you need microscope skills in Microbiology and Pathology. Nothing is more frustrating than being unable to "see anything" in your microscope while everyone else in the class seems to be looking at a whole new world.

Become so expert in using the microscope that it feels like second nature. This allows you to be very efficient in the laboratory exercises awaiting you. The point of these labs, after all, is to concentrate on the structures you are studying, not to worry about the details of using a microscope.

Using a word processing program on a computer – Once you know how to type, learn the rudiments of using a word processor. Word processors are computer programs that let you write, edit, spell-check, style, and print papers, reports, and even your "great American novel" if you are so inclined. Word processors are extremely valuable time-savers for writing the papers and reports that will be required of you.

As with typing programs, your medical school probably has word processing capability (and help learning how to use it) available for your use in the library or computer center. Make inquiries and get familiar with the programs open to you.

Writing/speaking skills – Throughout your career, it will be important for you to communicate by writing and by speaking. You will have to communicate your thoughts, ideas, and knowledge to your teachers, fellow students, preceptors, head residents, and patients and their families. It is especially important for you to be able to communicate effectively with your patients, often under circumstances where they are ill, frightened, don't wish to hear what you have to say, and are not especially knowledgeable about medicine. These are factors that will greatly detract from their ability to understand what you are trying to tell them. It is your duty to be as skillful as possible at communicating and overcome these barriers with your patients.

Practice explaining things to others at every opportunity. This may include explaining whatever you may be studying at the time to your spouse, a family member, loved one, or a fellow student. You may want to strike a bargain with another student, and agree to listen to each other's explanations. Do this regularly as a part of your study program. It will help you be sure you really understand what you are attempting to explain and help you remember it. The act of organizing and then explaining something is powerful active learning. You will probably learn from your colleague's explanations as well.

Chapter 7

Time Management

Why bother ? – The most important factors to successful study in medical school are effective organization and management of your time. High productivity in medical school requires careful, comprehensive planning.

Managing learning in medical school is no different from managing a complex business: high efficiency and high productivity are at a premium. To achieve this in the corporate world, upper-management professionals frequently receive extensive training in time and resource management. Similarly, the most successful medical students take a highly organized approach to life—carefully planning when they will study in relation to scheduled class time and other important life activities (e.g., eating, sleeping, exercising, family time, banking).

Have a life – There is absolutely no reason why a medical student cannot "have a life"—at least one evening per week to relax, one day per weekend free of academic concerns, and sufficient time to do the laundry, buy groceries, watch T.V., exercise, etc. This will depend on your ability to design and carry out a well thought-out study and life plan from the very first day of medical school. A *laissez faire*, I'll-wait-and-see-what-happens attitude could prove devastating. Avoid falling into a "catch-up trap" – a situation where you are constantly trying to catch-up, trying to second guess exam content, neglecting topics, or studying superficially and incompletely just to be (with some luck) minimally prepared for your exams.

Reduce stress – Some of the infamous stress commonly associated with the high-impact learning environment of medical school can be minimized by being organized at the outset. If you are well organized and on top of your studies, you can manage much better if something unforeseen occurs (e.g., illness, family problems, personal problems, unplanned social events).

Students who do not follow basic time-management principles frequently experience a sense of being "out of control" (i.e., the lectures, the material, the pace seem to dictate study patterns). Avoid this high-anxiety condition by being in control from the first day of medical school—get organized!

Enjoy spontaneity – If you are in control of your time, you can even afford to be spontaneous now and then; for example, going to the movies on the spur of the moment or taking time to visit with an unexpected guest. Being aware of your commitments and when you have scheduled free time, you can switch to an alternate time to accomplish what you had intended during an evening's study.

Designing an effective time-management plan – Designing an effective time-management plan requires that you have a complete schedule for each academic unit (e.g., semester, quarter, trimester, block) in your curriculum that includes all scheduled academic activities (e.g., lectures, labs, conferences, exams, electives) and all holidays.

The overview calendar – It is important to be fully aware of the most important commitments and time constraints you have during any academic unit. Buy a large calendar that allows you to view all the months of the first academic unit in a single glance and fill in your most critical and inflexible commitments as follows:

PERSONAL CALENDAR   MONTH: _October_

Sunday	Monday	Tuesday	Wednesday	Thursday	Friday	Saturday
					1	2
3	4	5	6	7	8 Biochem Exam (Krebs Cycle)	9
10 Tennis - Jack 12:30	11 Holiday No Class	12	13	14	15	16 Dentist 11:00
17	18	19	20 Histology Quiz (G.I. tract)	21	22	23 Diana's Wedding 2:30
24	25	26	27	28	29 Debbie's Halloween Party 9:00	30
31						

1. Mark in a bright color the dates and topics of all scheduled exams and quizzes.

2. Mark in a different color all scheduled holidays and study days.

3. Mark in a third color any important events in your own life that you plan to accommodate while in school (e.g., birthdays, weddings, reunions, religious observances, family events, important travel).

Place this calendar where you can see it daily and refer to it when necessary. Above your study desk is ideal.

Note carefully how your exams, study days, and important life commitments are spaced. Pay close attention to any pattern that will require special management, such as having several exams back-to-back, or a personal commitment that will interfere with studying just before an exam. Revise this overview calendar immediately if any schedule changes are announced or new inflexible personal commitments develop. (See the one-month sample overview calendar on the previous page.)

The weekly calendar – Make enough copies of the 24-hour, weekly time plan (on the next two pages) for each week of your semester. This will be your primary time-management plan and guide for each week. It should be comprehensive—anticipating not only when you will be in classes but also when you will accomplish life-maintenance activities, leisure activities, and, very importantly, studying.

Identify all weekly commitments – Before you begin to fill in this weekly planner, make a list of all your academic commitments for the week, all regular life-maintenance activities (e.g., eating, sleeping, food shopping), and all leisure activities that

- Academic activities
- Leisure and life activities
- Study time

WEEK OF: _____

TIME	MONDAY	TUESDAY	WEDNESDAY	THURSDAY	FRIDAY	SATURDAY	SUNDAY
7 AM							
8							
9							
10							
11							
12 PM							
1							
2							
3							
4							

Time	Monday	Tuesday	Wednesday	Thursday	Friday	Saturday	Sunday
5 PM							
6							
7							
8							
9							
10							
11							
12 AM							
1							
2							
3							
4							
5							
6							

you hope to retain (e.g., reading, exercise, T.V.). Plan your life and study hours around the inflexible academic commitments. Identify all commitments using the following categories and guidelines:

Academic activities – Have your syllabus and schedule for each ongoing course available.

Daily life-maintenance activities – These include sleeping, eating, traveling to and from school, etc.

Weekly life-maintenance activities – Make a list of all the important life-maintenance activities that you must take care of on a weekly basis. Think carefully and try to come up with a complete list. At a minimum this list should include things like food shopping, banking, laundry, housekeeping, and calling friends and family. You should also include religious observances, time commitments to children and/or your spouse, regular doctor's appointments, therapy sessions, etc. Put an asterisk next to any activity that must be scheduled at a specific predetermined time each week.

Leisure and social activities – Make a list of all the leisure and social activities that should be maintained while in medical school. These might include exercise, pleasure reading, television, visiting friends, etc. There is no reason why you should not be able to manage 5 to 7 hours of leisure activities per week. Participation in school clubs or student groups (e.g., student council, committees) should be included here. Put an asterisk next to activities that must be scheduled at a predetermined time (e.g., exercise class, meetings, favorite T.V. program).

Fill in the calendar – Follow the instructions below to construct your weekly calendar. Fill in each week using a different color for each numbered item. First, you should plan your academic and study schedule, then plan life-maintenance activities around these high-priority academic commitments. Finally, plan social and leisure activities around your study and life plan.

1. Fill in and label all scheduled academic activities for the week (e.g., lectures, labs, exams, electives). Be specific and include course names and subtopics.

2. Fill in all other rigidly scheduled activities (those marked with an asterisk in the above lists).

3. Now, plan the times you ideally will study each day of the week. Give yourself a minimum of four hours of study each day Monday through Friday for the first week and reserve another 6 to 8 hours for the weekend. You can add or delete study time in subsequent weeks according to your individual needs.

4. Look at the remaining items on your lists, and schedule time for each one. Consider using lunch breaks for things such as banking or business calls. Housekeeping, food shopping, and laundry may best be done on the weekends, but this will depend on your preference and how your school work is scheduled.

Weekly modifications as necessary – It is likely that most weeks will follow a similar pattern, however, it is advisable to reconsider your plan at the start of each week. In this way, you can regularly modify and adjust your routine to suit your own personal needs and accommodate any deviations from the routine in your classes. For example, the first week you may plan to study each weeknight from 7 to 11 PM, but after the first week you discover that you study more effectively in the morning from 6 to 8 AM and from 7 to 9 PM in the evening. You should feel free to modify your study plan to best suit your individual style and personality. Some people prefer to divide their study time into several small sessions of less than two hours each, while others prefer to study for longer periods at a single sitting. Some find late-night study most productive, others prefer early morning. In addition, changes in class time can occur and you should always be aware of these.

Implement the plan – The next step is to try to stick to your planned routine. It may be difficult to adjust and fine tune your schedule during the first week or two; but whatever you do, don't abandon your time-management plan. Like a new diet, an exercise program, or learning to drive a car, implementing a time-management plan can be a challenge. It requires hard work at the outset, but once it becomes automatic, it will result in a much better life-style.

Some basic principles – The following are some rules for good time management of your life during medical school:

1. Make a study-life plan and stick to it.

2. Find a regular place for study. If you find yourself constantly seeking a place that is "more conducive to focused study," reconsider the problem—is it the location or you? Self-discipline and resourcefulness (e.g., earplugs, answering machines, unplugged phones) are strategies that you should try.

3. If you deviate from your study routine, IMMEDIATELY plan when you will make up the topics that you had intended to study. Do not simply shift your entire plan back a day. This is not efficient and you will get farther and farther behind as the days go by. Instead, do your best to keep up with the material on a daily basis, returning to older unstudied material only if it is critical for an understanding of what you are currently studying.

4. Be completely up to date by the start of each new week. This means that you should have learned and memorized all the material from the prior week by the time you go to bed on Sunday night, "as if" you were going to be tested on Monday morning.

Special considerations for students with a spouse and/or children

Extra demands – Excellent time management and organizational skills are quintessential for students who must effectively juggle the demands of medical school, spouse, children, and running a household. Without such an approach, it is difficult to manage any, let alone all, of these demands in a relatively stress-free and efficient manner. The suggestions below should help you anticipate and manage some of the unique concerns that you may face.

Reassign tasks and learn to delegate – When considering all of your life-maintenance activities and family responsibilities, reassign as many as possible to your spouse, housekeeper, relatives, and/or baby-sitter. You must lighten your extracurricular load before you can add the heavy demands of being a successful student.

Involve your family – Involve your children and/or your spouse in the construction of your time plan. By sitting down together to work out your plan, all will be aware of the great demands that are placed on your time and energies. Be certain that everyone agrees and understands how important it is that you maintain this plan. Make certain that you enforce your study time and train your family that you must not be interrupted while you study.

Plan times with your partner – Don't forget that your spouse has a right to expect some time with you also. Plan regular times to socialize together. Much of the stress that can arise in relationships during medical school is due to the disappointment and frustration that results from repeatedly broken "dates." Avoid backing out of social plans with your partner at the last minute. Make it clear when you are and are not available, and plan times together that you definitely will be able to keep.

Post the plan for all to see – Post a copy of your time management plan in a place where it can easily be seen by your children, spouse, relatives, housekeeper, baby-sitter, and anyone else who depends on you. Use a special color for time with your children so they can see when they will have your undivided attention.

Be creative – You may need to get up extra early to maximize your study time. Learn to take a power nap (20 – 30 minutes) after the kids are in bed to refresh yourself before evening study. Plan to stay at school one or two evenings a week for intensive, high-yield study without interruptions.

Plan for exams – Review your examination schedule with your family and determine which weekends during the semester you will have to reduce family involvement to a minimum. Inform everyone and remind everyone regularly of these dates. Make some kind of exciting plan for the children on the weekends before exams. Doing this will reduce the likelihood that you will feel guilty and it will help keep your children from resenting your medical school commitments.

Keep everyone informed of changes – When your plans need revisions from time-to-time, be sure to keep everyone who counts on you fully informed. Let them know of any changes in your schedule as far in advance as possible.

Time Management

1. Find a regular **place** to study, where distractions and interruptions are minimized.

2. Plan regular **times** for **study**.

3. Plan regular **times** for **leisure**.

4. Plan **goals** for study **before** each study period in order of priority. Have specific goals for each 1/2 to 1-hour period.

5. Never stop studying in the middle of a topic. Take breaks at logical breaking points.

6. If unable to follow through on your study plan, plan catch-up study time immediately.

Chapter 8

Study Management

Introduction – Planning <u>when</u> you will study is the first step in designing a high-yield approach to medical school; planning just <u>what</u> to study is the next step. If you are to maximize your learning in the limited time you have, you should select what to study each day according to some basic rules of memory concepts. Memory has been studied extensively and one of the most widely accepted facts is that as soon as you are exposed to new information, you will gradually begin to forget it. The rate at which you forget, however, will be markedly influenced by just when you review and actualy attempt to commit the information to memory.

> Knowing what can affect memory should help you design the most efficient and effective study program.

Take advantage of short-term memory – Immediately after a lecture, lab, or small group activity, you will probably have about 70% to 80% recall of the information that was presented. Within 24 hours, without study, you will forget about half of that. You will forget even more if you did not understand the information particularly well. This forgetting can be minimized if you take advantage of the information while it is still in short-term memory by studying and learning it as soon as possible after class. Immediate review and memorization is the most time efficient way to study. If you wait just one day, it will take much longer to achieve the same level of mastery that can be achieved with immediate review.

Many students make a classic error when they get behind: in deciding what to study each day, they consider how easy the most recent material seems in relation to unstudied material from several days (weeks!) before. Inevitably, old material seems more difficult and is given study priority. The comparison is flawed, however, since it involves comparing information that has already undergone significant forgetting with information that is still fresh in your mind. If the recent material is neglected, it too will deteriorate and require more effort and time to learn when it is finally tackled.

Try to keep completely up to date by studying the most recent material on a daily basis. Each week, return to your time-management plan and fill in the content you expect to master each day to correspond with your syllabi.

To catch-up or to keep-up, that is the question – Occasionally, unforeseen events (i.e., illness, family commitments, free tickets to a new movie, a two-hour episode of your favorite television show, fatigue) can interfere with keeping up to date. If this occurs, it is important not to fall into the "catch-up" trap; abandoning the most recent material to try to master older, neglected material. Rather, only when you have mastered the current material, should you try to catch up. If you want to maximize your efficiency, never return to prior material unless it is essential to your understanding of the most recent material, and then limit your review to the specific sections of prior lectures that are critical. Most material can stand on its own, so think carefully before abandoning the most recent material for prior, unstudied material.

If you get behind, plan compensatory study immediately – The minute you get behind, you should plan when you will make-up the missed study. Review your time-management plan and reassign uncommitted study time or flexible leisure time to ensure that your studies are completely up to date by the beginning of each week. Remember that you will likely need extra time to learn material that has undergone forgetting. For example, if you need two to three hours to master a topic when it is studied as soon as possible after class, you will probably need three to four hours if study is postponed by more than a day.

Since it can take up to twice as long to master material that has undergone forgetting, the consequences of getting behind just one week can be overwhelming. Consider what can happen if the study accomplishments that ordinarily require about four hours of daily study are deferred and consequently require six hours to achieve the same level of mastery. First of all, over the course of five days, 20 hours of lost study becomes 30 hours of compensatory study. Trying to find 30 extra study hours over a weekend is not an appealing (or even reasonable) proposition. And it is even less reasonable to try and compensate during the following week when the 30 compensatory hours would need to be added onto the regular 20 hours for a total of 50 study hours. Since it rapidly becomes next to impossible to find enough time to make up for lost studies, students who get behind typically end up compromising the level of mastery and do not do as well on exams. Do your best to keep up to date, and catch-up as quickly as possible if you do get behind. (See Chapter 9 for further discussion of time-efficient, high-quality learning).

Learn and memorize on a daily basis – The goal of your studies is to transfer the information that you are learning in your courses to long-term memory. Basic science knowledge is the foundation of medicine. As a future physician, you must be able to recall many facts without hesitation. These facts will form the basis for much medical reasoning and problem solving in your basic science and clinical course work and as a practicing physician. Understanding concepts, principles, and mechanisms and "getting the gist of it" is a good beginning (in fact this is critical to effective learning, recall, and problem solving), but this is not enough—you must also regularly commit specific facts and details to memory.

Your ability to memorize effectively will depend on how well you understand the information and how you approach memorizing the facts and details. You should try to commit facts and details to memory on a daily basis, and not leave them until the last minute before exams. While cramming may have been an effective technique in undergraduate school, it is quite simply inappropriate in the rigorous medical school environment. Cramming breeds confusion and forgetting and rarely results in optimal performance on exams. Another hazard of cramming is that it rarely leads to good long-term retention of information. Don't forget that you will need to pass the United States Medical Licensing Examination (USMLE) in order to become licensed to practice medicine. The USMLE Step 1, addressing basic science, is typically taken at the end of your second year of medical school. This means that you must remember the information being taught to you well beyond the examinations within your current curriculum.

Daily memorization will make it easier to thoroughly master all your course work, and it will help you learn subsequent information more efficiently. For example, in Anatomy, if you first learn and memorize the positions and names of all the bones and bony processes in the upper limb, you will find it much easier to learn the names, locations, and functions of the muscles in the upper limb. Once you have learned the muscles, you will find it easier to memorize the nerves and blood supplies to these muscles. It is easier to learn new information when you have some related knowledge against which you can compare and contrast (see Chapter 10 on knowledge organization).

Minimize forgetting with intermittent review and self-testing – Even though you may learn and memorize information well today, it may still be subject to forgetting as the days and weeks progress. There are two useful methods to detect and compensate for this forgetting. The first is to intermittently review the information that you have mastered, the second is to test yourself regularly using old exams and practice questions.

Intermittent review – Intermittent review is critical for maintaining and transferring knowledge to long-term memory. Reviewing previously learned material is easy and very fast: what may have taken several hours to master initially, can be reviewed in just a few minutes. If you are keeping up to date, the weekend can provide an excellent opportunity to go over the material that you learned during the week. Another method of intermittent review is to spend 10 to 15 minutes reviewing material from the day before at the start of each daily study period. This gives you a chance to reinforce material and may serve to provide you with a better basis for learning any subsequent related material. Finally, you should take advantage of every opportunity to mentally review material that you have already learned. Your mind is like a muscle, it needs to be exercised to keep in shape. Think about the information that you are learning as frequently as possible—in the shower, while commuting, or even when walking between classes.

Intermittent Review Methods

• Use weekend study time to reinforce the material you studied and memorized during the week.

• Spend at least 10 to 15 minutes each day reviewing yesterday's material before you begin to study the material planned for today.

• Mentally recite and review material as often as is possible; in the shower, while commuting, while you are preparing meals, etc.

Self-testing – One of the greatest problems of forgetting is that it is difficult (if not impossible) to remember what has been forgotten. When mentally reviewing, you recite the information you remember, and omit what is forgotten without realizing it. Furthermore, reviewing from summaries or notes can lead to the false impression that you remember a lot, since memory is jogged by notes, and material that has been partially forgotten usually appears familiar. But familiarity and memory that is achieved through cued recall is not sufficient for solid performance on exams. One excellent method to help you identify topics that you have partially forgotten (or inadequately learned) is to use exams from previous years, practice questions from published review books, or study guides as an integral and regular part of your study.

If you use practice questions several days after you have completed study of a specific topic, you will be able to identify details that you have forgotten or concepts that you did not fully understand. You can then return to your notes and focus additional study on the knowledge gaps that you have discovered. It is important to wait several days after studying a topic before self-testing if you intend to find out what you have forgotten. Reviewing questions immediately after you study a topic can serve to help solidify your knowledge, but using short-term memories that can rapidly fade, may lead to an inflated estimate of how well you know the material.

Another benefit of using old exams and practice questions is that it helps students develop a sense of the level of detail and question types that they can expect to see on exams. Waiting until the day before an examination to look at old exams is of little value. What is the point of finding out what you don't know, or that you have misjudged the difficulty level of the exam when there is not enough time to do anything about it? Many students assume that the only reason to use practice questions is to find out if they "know enough to pass," and therefore they defer using the exams until they have completed their study. In fact, a more important use of old exams is to find out what you don't know while there is still time to do something about it!

Another method of self-testing is to find a studymate with whom you can spend time quizzing one another. The very exercise of formulating a good question for your study partner is a good method of intermittent review, and attempting to answer the questions of your studymate is an excellent way to identify areas that you may have failed to recognize as important.

Student note service – Many schools have a student-run note service in which summaries or transcripts of lectures are produced. Typically, lectures are audiotaped, and students are hired as scribes to make complete and accurate note sets. These are then copied and circulated to all students who subscribe to the service. There is wide variation from school to school and year to year in the quality, and therefore in the potential benefit, of these services. Carefully consider the issues below before deciding whether or not to subscribe to a note service. If the note service in your school is inadequate, then consider the structure of the optimal note service as described below and work with your fellow students and interested faculty to improve the system at your institution.

Problems with note services – Some of the greatest problems with note services are:

Timing – It usually takes three to five days for a note set to be circulated. This is enormously problematic since high-efficiency learning must be done the same day that one is exposed to the material (see Chapter 8 on study management and memory). If a student always waits to get the note sets before serious study of a topic, he or she will always take longer to learn the material and will likely resort to superficial study. A note service should only be used as a back-up system if it is not available immediately. Never use a note service as a substitute for lecture attendance.

Accuracy – Since lecturers can make mistakes, and student scribes can make mistakes—note service notes can be notoriously inaccurate. Without a thorough editing process, you must always be suspect of the accuracy of the note set. In some institutions however, faculty are willing to review, edit, and approve transcripts before distribution. If the notes are edited by faculty, they are much more reliable as a back-up resource.

Quality – Some students produce excellent, well-organized summaries, while others produce list-like incomprehensible summaries (see Chapter 10 on knowledge organization). A summary that is considered great by one student may be lousy from the perspective of another. For example, some students love charts, while others prefer more elaborated summaries. One person likes pictures, another prefers words. There is quite simply no guarantee that the note sets will be high quality or be of an optimal format for your own personal learning style.

The best note services – The best student note services are characterized by:

Last year's notes – They provide one-sided copies of last year's notes to all students at the start of each year (unless your school has just undergone a comprehensive curriculum revision, 80% to 90% of the material will likely be the same). Last year's notes can be a highly efficient source for: (1) preparing for lectures, (2) taking additional notes on the blank pages during lectures, and (3) reviewing after lecture.

Computer-based – They are computer-based, so that the scribe's job is to improve upon the note sets from prior years instead of reinventing the wheel each year. The scribe should be responsible for producing a summary of any significant changes (e.g., errors, omissions, additions) from prior years' notes.

Faculty support – They have the approval and editing support of the faculty. It is unlikely that faculty will approve of a note service unless it complies with the first two conditions in this list, and is not used as a substitute for lecture attendance.

Memorization Techniques

• Use old exams and practice questions at least once a week to identify information that you have forgotten or did not learn well in the first place.

• Wait several days before self-testing to allow forgetting-prone topics to surface.

• Quiz and be quizzed by your friends and members of your study group.

• Don't wait until the day before an exam to use old exams; find out what you don't know in time to compensate with additional study.

The Amount to be Gained by Study

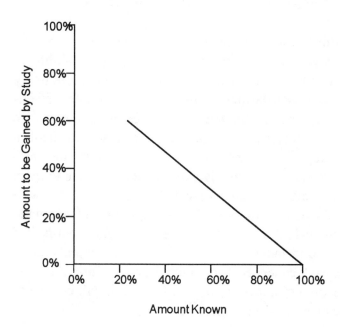

This figure illustrates that you will gain far more by studying those subjects about which you know the least. Be selective in what you choose to study, especially when time is short.

Chapter 9

Getting the Most Out of Your Classes

Introduction – Taking the time to prepare for lectures, labs, and conferences can have a dramatic impact on your ability to understand and learn from these activities. This preliminary work does not need to be time intensive: 15 to 30 minutes of well-organized preparation should be effective. Even lectures that are regarded as "poor" can be significantly enhanced through a structured preparation. The goal is not to learn all the information ahead of time or to merely skim the topics – it is to learn about the organization of the topic, to become acquainted with the most important terminology, and to begin to think about the potential clinical relevance of the material. In other words, it is to develop a solid understanding of "the big picture" and knowledge of the basic concepts. The better your preparation, the more you will get out of a lecture, and the faster you will be able to master the material after the lecture.

Anyone who has ever attended an opera or a ballet without reading the synopsis beforehand will fully appreciate the potential benefits of a simple preparation. A synopsis provides an overview of the story line, introduces the names of the key characters, and enables the audience to interpret more fully the details of the story even when it is performed in a foreign language (Italian, dance, etc.). Failure to read the synopsis can result in confusion, the false perception that the opera has little if any story line, and early nodding off. Similarly, anyone who has watched a tennis match without knowing the basic rules of the game and the background of the players' strengths and weaknesses is at a serious disadvantage for enjoyment of the game. The same phenomenon applies to academics, where failing to prepare for lectures (or labs, or conferences) can result in confusion, poor note taking, and a greater risk of tuning out.

A solid preparation for lectures should result in better note taking, a greater interest in the material, and more active listening. If you get more out of your lectures, you will need less time to learn and memorize the material afterward. Similarly, if you are well prepared for labs, you will be more efficient and productive during the lab, and take less time to master the material. An informal survey of medical students who were elected to Alpha Omega Alpha revealed that over 80% always attended lectures, and always prepared beforehand.

Lecture preparation – The primary goal of lecture preparation is to develop a solid understanding of the organization of the material that is to be presented and to learn some of the basic vocabulary, terminology, and concepts. You will know if you achieved this by asking yourself the following two simple questions after the lecture:

1. Did I have a "table of contents" in my head that allowed me to anticipate the general progression of the topics of the lecture? (Good preparation = YES)

2. Did I find myself trying to write down words and definitions so that I was distracted from the meaning of the lecture? (Good preparation = NO)

Find a good reference – The first step is to identify a good source in which the organization of the material is well highlighted through section titles, headings, and subheadings. Furthermore, a source that includes detailed diagrams, charts, or other visual aids can be most helpful. Review your syllabus, textbooks, review books, and old transcripts (or class notes) and select the one that is the best organized. You should consult your syllabus to verify that your selected source covers all the material. You may need to change your preparation source now and then if the quality varies from section to section.

Read the objectives, introduction, conclusion, and any summary remarks – Once you have identified your source, the next step is to read any objectives that are provided in your syllabus or preparation source. If there are none, read the introductory paragraphs, the concluding paragraphs, and any summary remarks. Do not skip over the introductory comments – they are the best way for you to begin developing an understanding of the "big picture."

Make an outline of the material with major headings and subheadings –The next step is to develop a "table of contents" for the lecture. This is often provided in the course syllabus. However, it may require that you leaf through your study source and excerpt (or create) major headings and subheadings as if preparing an outline for the lecture. Some textbooks provide such a topical outline at the start of each chapter. (*Pathology*, by Robbins, is an excellent example of such a text.) As you make this content outline, you should be noting several of the following things about each section:

  How much space is devoted to each section? – Sections that cover several pages are likely to be more important and possibly more difficult than topics that receive shorter coverage.

  How difficult and/or detailed does each section appear? – It is wise to identify subtopics that appear to be particularly difficult or complex and to be certain to pay full attention when that material is being addressed in the lecture.

How familiar is the material in each section? – You will have covered some topics as an undergraduate, others will be completely new. For familiar topics, ask yourself if the level of detail is greater than your expectation. For new topics, make a note to pay close attention during a lecture and prepare a list of basic vocabulary items.

How does this topic relate to topics previously covered in the course? – As the year progresses, you will be able to integrate information from one section of a course to another and also across courses. For example, in Biochemistry as you progress through different metabolic pathways, you will learn that some biochemical reactions take place in the mitochondria, while others occur in the cytosol. You should always be striving to identify this kind of relationship across sections.

What is the potential clinical relevance of this material? – Raising questions about the potential clinical relevance of basic science material can help you keep it in perspective and heighten your level of interest. For example, when confronted with learning a cross-section of the neck, you might raise questions about the appropriate surgical routes of entry to various structures, or think about the damage that could occur with bullet wounds entering at different angles and locations.

Skim your source to get the gist of it – Only after you have a clear and well-organized lecture outline in your head should you skim the notes or chapter. This should be done very quickly, merely scanning each section to identify terms that seem to frequently recur. If you are very short on time, this is the one step that can be omitted, since you will have done some skimming to answer the questions raised in the previous section.

Read and learn definitions for basic vocabulary and concepts – The next step is to read and define all terms that are listed in boldface, italics, or otherwise highlighted. If your source does not have some form of highlighting, make an effort to skim the material and pull out major content words that occur frequently or seem to be central to the topic. Know as many of these definitions as possible before going to the lecture. There is nothing more discouraging than finding yourself unable to follow the lecture because you are at the level of learning basic definitions while the lecture is elaborating and relating these concepts in complex ways. Below are some examples of the types of learning and memorizing that can be done before a lecture or lab in several different basic Science courses. Pay careful attention to when memorization is specified in a preparation, and when merely mentally remarking is sufficient.

Anatomy – Upper limb: Memorize the names and positions of the bones and bony processes in the region of your dissection before lab. Make a list of the muscles' names and functions separately. List the nerves separately. Locate each structure in your atlas.

Biochemistry – Metabolic pathways: Memorize the names of the major substances in the order of their occurrence in the biochemical pathway. Note the structural differences between these substances in very basic terms (e.g., 5 carbons vs. 6 carbons; phosphate group vs. no phosphate group). Memorize the names of enzymes and cofactors. Identify energy requirements. Note if the location of the reaction (e.g., mitochondria) is relevant.

Physiology – Renal: Memorize the names and general functions of each part of the kidney. Memorize the names and general functions of each part of the nephron. Note to what degree histology is reviewed or discussed. Note the ions that are exchanged at different locations in the nephron.

Pathology – Memorize the names of related diseases, and memorize one important dimension of the pathology (gross pathology or histopathology) for each one.

Pharmacology – Antiseizure drugs: Memorize the major classes of mechanisms by which anticonvulsants control seizures and learn the drug names in each class. Review the major types of seizures.

Preview diagrams, graphs, pictures, charts, etc. – Look at any pictures, graphs, diagrams, or other visual summaries that are in your syllabus, note sets, and text. Read the caption for each and think briefly about how each one relates to the content outline that you have prepared. Frequently, instructors will use the same visuals as slides or overheads; if you familiarize yourself with what is in your study sources ahead of time, you will minimize frantic note-taking and you can sit back and pay attention to the discussion of the material. The *MedCharts* series of books contains summaries of course material in chart, graph, and tabular form. See:

Rosenbach, K.P., *Pharmacology: MedCharts*, Granville, OH, ILOC, 1993.

Gest, T., *Anatomy: MedCharts*, Granville, OH, ILOC, 1994.

Laboratory preparation – Laboratory preparation is just as important as lecture preparation and possibly more so. In lectures, you are responsible only to yourself, but labs are typically group activities. Being unprepared for a lab could be detrimental to your entire group if you cannot pull your weight. In addition, lack of preparation can breed feelings of inadequacy when other group members come prepared and can progress rapidly utilizing information they learned ahead of time.

A solid preparation for a lab should include a thorough understanding of the objectives. These are usually provided in the laboratory manual. It is important to be clearly aware of the content objectives of the lab, and much less important to be aware of specific lab procedures. (Note any procedures where safety is an issue or that are critical to the outcome of the lab– these are usually highlighted or clearly defined by lab directors.) In your own mind, however, you should separate the content of the lab from the methods. Place your emphasis for study and remembering on the content.

Just as with lectures, it can be helpful to try to memorize a few of the most basic facts before a lab.

Benefits of Laboratory Preparation

1. Greater efficiency during the lab (i.e., saves time).

2. Increases learning that takes place during the lab.

3. Increases long-term retention of information.

4. Reduces postlaboratory learning time.

Preparation for conferences, small groups, problem solving sessions, etc. – Small group activities such as these are of little benefit without comprehensive preparation. In contrast to lectures and labs where overviews and learning basic vocabulary are sufficient as a preparation, small group activities are usually designed to elaborate on well-established knowledge. Most small group teaching activities require students to apply their knowledge to problems, answer questions, and participate in discussions. It is impossible to do any of these unless all assigned readings, all practice problems, and all prior-related lecture material has been mastered to the best of your ability. Another purpose of small groups is to help students resolve difficult concepts; so don't despair if you have not completely mastered the material before a small group activity. If you have done your best, but some questions still remain, you can take advantage of small groups to improve your understanding.

Learning in a clinical environment – When you move from the basic sciences into the clinical sciences, you progress from a highly structured and planned learning environment into one that is much less rigid. Your days are primarily spent on hospital wards with patients, and lectures are reduced to a minimum. Much of your learning is structured around the specific patients that you are helping to admit and manage. But if you limit study and learning to the specifics of your patients' problems, you may do very well clinically but you won't be learning enough to prepare yourself to pass the USMLE Step 2 examination or comprehensive written examinations required in your clinical courses. You need to read extensively to be certain that your learning is comprehensive. In the same way that you must develop a well-integrated and organized foundation in the basic sciences, you must do the same in your clinical years.

Make a time management plan for study – Time management and planning are as critical in the clinical years as they are in the basic science years. Review your syllabus for each clinical course and plan regular study times according to the guidelines in Chapter 8. Make sure that you include enough time to read and study all areas that are outlined in your syllabus. The order in which you review specific subtopics in each clinical course (e.g., respiratory, renal, cardiovascular) is less important than planning enough time to thoroughly study each area.

Keep track of the big picture – You may find it useful to consider each patient's primary problem as an entry point into a specific field of clinical medicine. For example, if you have been assigned a patient with myocardial infarction, use this as a window into ischemic heart disease, and more broadly, into cardiovascular medicine. It's easier and more interesting to learn about other types of cardiovascular disease if you have a relationship with a real clinical case. Important similarities and differences among various disorders of the cardiovascular system emerge and are more easily learned.

Study the differential diagnoses – For each patient that you encounter, you need to understand the diagnostic process (e.g., history, physical exam, lab tests) that enables the attending physician to converge upon a set of potential diagnoses and to then select the best diagnosis from among the set of possibilities. Be certain that you understand why the differential diagnoses were initially identified, and then how and why each one was ruled out. If you take the time to read comprehensively about each diagnosis that you encounter, it will be easier for you to develop an organized mental filing system that will enable you to learn and to problem-solve most effectively.

Use practice questions – There are several publications that provide well-edited, typically organized USMLE-type practice questions for each clinical science. These collections of questions provide an excellent study source for USMLE Step 2 (see the section on self-evaluation in Chapter 8).

Chapter 10

Knowledge Organization

Introduction – Your ability to acquire knowledge efficiently and effectively goes beyond careful preparation and well-structured study time; an active approach to learning is also required. How you summarize and organize the information that you are learning has a dramatic impact on your ability to memorize, retain, and later use that information. You must be an active participant in the learning process, and not just a passive recipient of information.

A tremendous number of facts and concepts are presented in lectures, texts, and labs. Studies have shown that how this information is organized in the memory is quite different for high-performing medical students in relation to lower performing medical students. High-performers integrate material so that it is logically organized to highlight important relationships. Weaker students are more likely to present information as poorly organized lists without clearly illustrating logical relationships.

Integrate and organize – To maximize your ability to learn, recall, and apply facts and concepts to problem-solving situations, you must integrate and organize them in your mind for easy retrieval. In essence, you need to create a thoroughly cross-referenced "mental" filing system of both basic science and clinical information.

Some lecturers present information in a, well-organized manner, moving from general principles to specific examples.

Throughout their lectures, they take the time to highlight important relationships, similarities, and differences between the topics they are currently discussing and ones that have been encountered elsewhere. Other lecturers explain the specific topic of the day, and leave the task of optimally organizing the information to the student.

The first step in organizing the information you encounter is to prepare for lectures and labs as described in Chapter 9. This preparation is designed to give you a framework for the material you are learning. The next step is to elaborate this framework to create a concise, integrated, accurate summary of all the facts and concepts. This requires an active approach to learning.

Passive learning is ineffective – Many students are overwhelmed by the sheer volume of information that must be mastered in medical school and lapse into any one of a variety of passive-study approaches. In some cases, this involves nothing more than rote memorization of facts. In other cases, it consists of reading, re-reading, and re-re-reading the same material. It may involve rewriting note sets in much the same way that the information is presented in the lecture or text. Or it may entail highlighting to the point of creating a "jaundiced" or "psychedelic" text or note set. These approaches may give the impression of being comprehensive and efficient, but they rarely result in adequate learning. Studies of learning and memory have demonstrated that repeated exposure is not an effective method for transferring information into long-term memory:

Nickerson, R.S. & Adams, M.J. (1979). Long-term memory for a common object. *Cognitive Psychology* 11: 287-307.

The American Nickel – You have looked at the head side of this coin many, many times, but can you answer the following questions? (DON'T LOOK AT A REAL NICKEL YET.)

1. Who's profile is featured on the nickel?

2. Which direction does the profile face?

3. What words are written on the head side?

4. What is the location of any print on the head side?

Most people have great difficulty answering more than one or two of these questions with accuracy or confidence. Occasionally, people respond to this challenge by saying that although they have difficulty recalling this level of detail, they could certainly recognize a nickel. See if you can recognize the nickel in the group of sketches below.

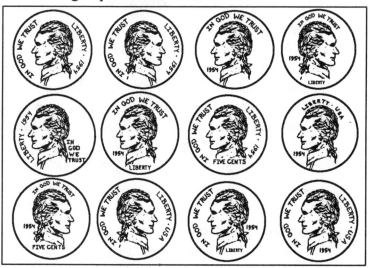

Even in the context of a multiple-choice question, it is difficult to identify the correct picture. Clearly, repeated viewing does not result in good recall or recognition.

Active learning – If repetition does not lead to a sufficient level of learning, what kind of study approach does? Active learning. This involves:

- Putting information into your own words.

- Reorganizing information when necessary to high-light similarities and differences between concepts.

- Making (or using) charts, flow diagrams, schematic diagrams, and other kinds of summaries that highlight important comparisons and contrasts, and that allow you to integrate information.

- Keeping track of the BIG PICTURE and organiza-tional principles at all times.

- Highlighting in a very selective way.

How to learn the details – Let's return to the nickel and con-sider how to best go about learning the details. One approach is to study the nickel and rotely memorize all of its details. This approach will undoubtedly enable you to answer all of the previous questions, but how would you fare, if after memorizing the nickel, you were asked to answer similar questions about a penny or a dime? It is unlikely that you would have much success with these other coins based on your study of the nickel.

Now consider an alternative, more active, approach to learn-ing about the nickel that involves comparing and contrasting it with other American coins (i.e., a penny, a dime, a quarter, and a fifty-cent piece). If you did this, you would discover some important similarities and differences about coins—in other words, some rules about coins:

RULE 1: On the head side of every American coin there are three, and only three, items that appear (other than the picture): the year (e.g., 1976); the phrase *In God We Trust*, and the word *Liberty*.

Return to the nickels and eliminate all of the alternatives that do not satisfy this rule.

RULE 2: On all coins, with the exception of the penny, the profile of the head faces to the left.

With just these two rules, you can eliminate eight of the twelve options in the multiple choice version of the question. Furthermore, you could eliminate the same number of options if asked about a penny, a dime, or a quarter. Comparing and contrasting allows you detect redundancies and exceptions that facilitate learning and problem solving. In addition, the grouping of facts according to similarities reduces the load on memory and makes memorization easier.

RULE 3: The exact location of the printed words and the year is different for each coin.

This third rule of American coins captures the next stage in the learning process—the identification of details that must be memorized to converge on the exact answer to a question. You must memorize the exact location of each printed item on the nickel (and the name of the president who is featured on it). If you master the details of the nickel before trying to tackle any other coin, you discover that it is easier to learn the details of the other coins.

(IT IS OK TO LOOK AT A REAL NICKEL NOW.)

A problem-solving question – Let's consider the following problem-solving question:

> The United States has decided to mint a new seventy-five-cent coin. Please design your version of the head side for this new coin.

Knowing the rules of coins that are listed above and the details of each existing coin, you are able to design this new coin with ease. In contrast, an approach that focused on learning only the details of each existing coin would render this activity extremely challenging if not altogether impossible.

How memory works – If you have taken the time to work through this example, not only have you learned about American coins, but you have also gained important insight into how memory most easily works; through encoding relationships (similarities and differences) in a logical, organized manner and moving from the generalities (the BIG PICTURE), to the specifics (filling in the details and exceptions to the rules). You should approach learning in every one of your courses in this way.

Implementing an active study approach in a time-efficient manner –Many students recognize the value of active study strategies, but reject them for more superficial passive strategies because of the time element. Some students argue that active strategies that involve the reorganization of information are too time consuming. But the facts are clear—without an active approach, it is unlikely that you can master the material at an adequate level to perform well on exams. Remember that while active strategies such as making summaries, charts, etc., may be more time consuming at the outset, they save time in the long run. A well-organized summary enables you to memorize and efficiently learn in greater detail, and provides an expedient source for highly efficient review just before examinations. The more you practice active approaches to learning, the faster you become at implementing them.

Taking advantage of summaries – You should take advantage of summaries that appear in handouts, texts, and review books. Creating your own summary yields the best learning (if it is well organized), but it can sometimes be more efficient to use summaries that others have already created. You may find it useful to borrow the structure of a summary from a text or review book, and then to fill in the details on your own.

Demonstrations of active approaches to summarizing – In the sections that follow, we have provided some examples of how to structure effective, well-organized summaries in various subject areas. The optimal form of a summary depends on the subject matter and the level of detail in which it is presented.

The first example shows how to use text or note-set margins to outline topic headings that can be used to guide highlighting, and to provide the basic headings for a summary chart. The passage in this example is used with permission from:

Kingsbury, D.T. et al., *The National Medical Series for Independent Study: Microbiology,* Media, Pa, Harwal Publishing Company, 1985.

Highlighting and outlining – Try your hand at outlining and highlighting the passage on treatment for MYCOSES (i.e., fungal infections) on the next page.

MYCOSES

D. THERAPY – Several antifungal agents play unique roles in the treatment of serious fungal infections. Whatever their apparent *in vitro* effects, the antifungals tend to behave as fungistatic drugs *in vivo*, a fact that emphasizes the importance of host defenses in successful recovery from systemic fungal infection.

1. Amphotericin B is a polyene antibiotic that binds to ergosterol in the outer membrane of fungi, thus increasing cell permeability. It is given parenterally, and limitations in dosage are imposed by its multiple (especially renal) toxicities. The spectrum of activity includes most of the systemic fungal pathogens.

2. 5-Fluorocytosine (5-FC) is a compound metabolized to 5-fluorouracil (5-FU) in fungal cells, thus interfering with fungal RNA synthesis. 5-FC is clinically useful only against yeasts. Although it may be used as an oral agent, it must be used in combination with other antifungals because of the rapid development of resistant mutants when 5-FC is used alone.

3. Imidazole compounds probably act by interfering with ergosterol synthesis, thus affecting membrane permeability. Clinically useful antifungal agents from this group include ketoconazole, an oral agent with activity against a number of yeasts and dimorphic fungi, and miconazole, which is available in parenteral and topical preparations.

4. Nystatin, a polyene antibiotic, is used for topical applications.

Try to design a good summary and write it below.

When you are finished – Now that you are finished, consider our approach to this passage of text.

Note topic headings in the margins – Compare your notations and highlighting to the ones we have illustrated on the next page. The margin notes are topic categories that are used to direct the highlighting.

MYCOSES

D. THERAPY – Several antifungal agents play unique roles in the treatment of serious fungal infections. Whatever their apparent *in vitro* effects, the antifungals tend to behave as fungistatic drugs *in vivo,* a fact that emphasizes the importance of host defenses in successful recovery from systemic fungal infection.

4 main ones

1. **Amphotericin B** is a polyene antibiotic that binds to ergosterol in the outer membrane of fungi, thus increasing cell permeability. It is given parenterally, and limitations in dosage are imposed by its multiple (especially renal) toxicities. The spectrum of activity includes most of the systemic fungal pathogens.

1. Drug Class
2. Mechanism
3. Administration
4. Side Effects
5. Spectrum

2. **5-Fluorocytosine** (5-FC) is a compound metabolized to 5-fluorouracil (5-FU) in fungal cells, thus interfering with fungal RNA synthesis. 5-FC is clinically useful only against yeasts. Although it may be used as an oral agent, it must be used in combination with other antifungals because of the rapid development of resistant mutants when 5-FC is used alone.

3. **Imidazole compounds** probably act by interfering with ergosterol synthesis, thus affecting membrane permeability. Clinically useful antifungal agents from this group include ketoconazole, an oral agent with activity against a number of yeasts and dimorphic fungi, and miconazole, which is available in parenteral and topical preparations.

examples

4. **Nystatin,** a polyene antibiotic, is used for topical applications.

Are Side Effects same as Amphotericin B?
Is Mechanism same as " "?
Spectrum ?

How to do it – The procedure to construct the highlighting:

1. An overview of the entire passage and a reading of the introductory statement identified the "4 main" Mycoses therapies that are noted in the margin, and that "host defenses" (highlighted) contribute to the ability to fight fungal infections.

2. Reading the entire first statement on Amphotericin B revealed five important categories of information that were presented in the passage as noted in the margin: (1) Drug Class; (2) Mechanism of Action; (3) Route of Administration; (4) Side Effects; and (5) Spectrum of Action.

3. After these five categories were identified, highlighting was numbered and limited to the key words that provided the specific details for each category of information.

4. Reading the entire second statement on 5-fluorocytosine revealed, in a slightly different order, all of the same categories of information that were presented for amphotericin B, with the exception of the drug class. The same was true for the third statement on imidazole compounds. Therefore, the key words in each paragraph were highlighted and numbered accordingly.

5. The last paragraph appeared, at first glance, to contain only two pieces of information. However, an active approach to study would immediately detect the similarity between nystatin and amphotericin B—they are both polyene antibiotics. As an active learner, you should ask yourself if the mechanisms and side effects are the same. Also, since nystatin is administered topically rather than parenterally, it is not likely to be used for systemic infections (as is amphotericin B).

Key words – Pay close attention to how only key words are highlighted. When you return to this passage, if the highlighted words fail to trigger more complete memories, you have not adequately learned this material.

Making a summary chart – The recurring margin headings become the column headings for a summary chart. The underlined words become the basis for details that are entered in each cell. Notice the following advantages of the chart summary:

1. Charts highlight similarities and differences among the ideas. For example, note that three of the drugs have similar mechanisms of action (i.e., affect cell permeability through ergosterol), and two are polyene antibiotics. Each grouping makes it easier to memorize and to later retrieve.

2. Note that not every cell is filled in; "?" was entered when specific information was not provided or was entered through inference. This allows you to detect missing information, or information that may require verification.

3. Abbreviations and symbols have been used to economize space, time, and effort.

The optimal form of a summary depends upon the subject matter – The optimal form of a summary depends to some extent on the nature of the material that is being summarized. For example, Anatomy is best summarized through schematic drawings that are supplemented with charts; Biochemistry and Physiology tend to require flow charts and graphic summaries; Pharmacology, Microbiology, and Pathology are well suited for charts. Regardless of the specific form of the relational summaries that you use, they should all meet the following important general standards:

Overview of Treatment for Mycoses Infections

Drug Name	Drug Class	Mechanism	Administration	Side Effects	Spectrum
amphotericin B	polyene antibiotic	binds ergosterol ↑ permeability	parenteral	renal toxicities	systemic
5-fluorocytosine	?	interferes with RNA synthesis	oral	resistant mutants	yeasts
imidazole	e.g., ketoconaz. ---- miconaz.	interferes ergosterol synth. ↑ permeability	oral ---- parenteral topical	?	yeasts dimorphic ---- ?
nystatin	polyene antibiotic	binds ergosterol ↑ permeability	topical	?	?

1. Every summary should have a title.

2. A good summary is organized by general categories, or dimensions, along which details are organized. For example, a chart summarizing the muscles of an extremity should have the following categories for each muscle in the region: origin, insertion, function, nerve supply, and blood supply. In Biochemistry, a chart or flow diagram for a metabolic pathway should include: structures, substrate names, enzymes (reaction type), cofactors, energy requirements, by-products, and location of reaction. In Pharmacology, charts should include the following categories: drug name, mechanism of action, therapeutic use, route of administration, pharmacodynamics (distribution, half-life, clearance), and side effects.

3. A good summary visually highlights (i.e., in a single glance) important comparisons and contrasts within a category (i.e., it should be easy to see which muscles have the same functions, which have the same innervations, etc.).

4. A good summary uses very few words and makes effective use of standard abbreviations.

5. A good summary is complete and accurate.

Organizing information in Anatomy – Anatomy is a visual-spatial science that is usually taught through direct study of the three-dimensional structures and their "geography." Since dissection is done regionally, it is sometimes difficult to visualize long-distance relationships such as nerve and arterial pathways. Excellent integrated summaries are important tools in organizing anatomical information. Since Anatomy is primarily visual, your summaries should include schematic drawings and diagrams of structures and the relationships among the structures.

It's helpful to memorize the names and locations of bones as the first step in the learning process; this provides you with a framework of reference for mapping on muscles, organs, nerves, and blood supplies. Later, additional details can be superimposed on this knowledge base.

You may find it useful to supplement schematic drawings with charts that summarize important similarities and differences among structures. For example, muscles can be grouped by region, function, nerve supply, and blood supply. A chart that lists all the muscles in the posterior forearm will reveal that they are all innervated by the radial nerve. It is much easier to learn this generalization before beginning a dissection, otherwise it may be overlooked or only emerge after much time and effort is spent memorizing individual muscles and their innervations.

Organizing information in Physiology – The optimal summary format in Physiology will vary considerably from topic to topic. Flow diagrams that summarize the sequences of events, and mechanisms of control in a physiological process, graphs and equations that show quantitative relationships, and charts all prove to be useful summary forms as you master Physiology. Use your textbook and other resources to identify summaries that integrate and highlight relationships.

Organizing information in Biochemistry – Flow charts are excellent for summarizing metabolic pathways. When you create a flow chart, don't try to fill in all the details of each step in the pathway from the beginning to the end. Instead, start by summarizing the sequence of structural changes (and biochemical names) at each step in the pathway. In other words, look at what you are starting with, what you end up with, and what structural changes occur to get you from the first step to your product. Once you have mastered (memorized) the structural pathway, then map on the enzymatic requirements for the various steps. Energy requirements can be added next, followed by other important categories of information such as by-products, location of the reaction, etc.

Organizing information in Microanatomy and Pathology – In general, both of these subjects lend themselves to a combination of schematic drawings and chart form.

Organizing information in Microbiology and Pharmacology – In general, both of these subjects can be best summarized in charts.

Putting it all together – At this stage, you have read about how to design a high-yield program that organizes your life and studies, effectively prepares you for academic activities and how to study in an active manner that should result in an elaborate, well-organized, and integrated mental filing system of basic science and medical information. We have summarized the study recommendations of a group of students who performed at the highest level in Anatomy, and another group who performed at the highest level in Biochemistry. We selected these two subjects, since they are apt to be encountered early in medical school. Note that each set of recommendations follows all the guidelines that you have read about up to this point.

Anatomy Guidelines

1. Prepare for labs and lectures by

• reading the objectives.

• familiarizing yourself with all of the structures to be dissected and specific relevant topics.

• listing all of the structures you will be expected to find during the laboratory session.

2. Draw sketches to highlight relationships. Try to draw from memory.

3. Go to the lab at least one extra time each week with another person and quiz each other.

4. Learn (memorize) as much as you can every day. Constantly review previous material, so that new material is added onto a base of information.

5. Read old examination questions each week to know the base of information (i.e., the general emphasis, the level of detail, and the format of questions) that is expected. Do not wait until the last minute to do this.

6. Do any problem sets and read through and understand all clinical correlations in the textbook. Make sure you have studied and tried to learn all the relevant information first.

7. Take electives, if possible, since they often teach you relationships.

8. Use cross-sections and x-rays of the anatomy to help learn relationships.

Biochemistry Guidelines

1. Prepare for lectures from handouts (or texts, or syllabi) to get the main idea.

2. Get the main idea first. After the lecture, learn more specific details. Always remind yourself of the basic concepts that are being presented.

3. Memorize one structure and know the permutations that result in different but related structures.

4. Draw out the pathways: first draw structures and names, next add enzymes, then cofactors, then energy, etc.

5. Learn similarities and differences between pathways (i.e., compare and contrast purine and pyrimidine synthesis and catabolism).

6. Make a huge flow chart for metabolic integration:

• half in the cytosol, half in the mitochondria.

• include: glycolysis, hexosemonophosphate shunt, Krebs cycle, oxidative phosphorylation, fatty acid synthesis and breakdown, amino acid metabolism, and nitrogen metabolism.

• pay attention to the role of coenzymes and cofactors (i.e., vitamins and minerals).

• note energy pumps, protein channels, and shuttle proteins.

7. Chart (or draw a picture of) hormones and second messenger mechanisms.

Chapter 11

Stress Management
by Janice N. McLean, Ph.D.
Denison University and

Private Practice in Clinical Psychology

Congratulations! – You have converted your dream of becoming a doctor into a reality. You are in medical school preparing for one of life's most difficult, challenging, and rewarding careers. One part of this new challenge is to meet responsibility with the least possible psychological stress, a seemingly difficult task given the enormity of the medical school curriculum. The purpose of this chapter is to help you do just that.

First, let's clarify what is meant by the term psychological stress. By definition, psychological stress is the result of a relationship between a person and the environment, in which the person believes the situation is overwhelming and threatens his or her ability to cope. This situation may be one that is generally validated by all as a stressful one, for example, being approached by a mugger, or one that seems less universally threatening, such as getting a C on an important exam.

General adaptation syndrome – When a person views an event or situation as stressful, the body reacts by initiating the fight or flight response. Physician Hans Selye defined this as the general adaptation syndrome. This syndrome prepares the body to fight the stressor or to run away from it. As a child, the threatening neighborhood bully may have evoked the fight or flight response in you. Seeing him (her?), your immediate thought would be — "Uh-oh! I'm in danger from . . . " Accordingly, the body would respond to this cognitive perception by preparing you to either fight with or to run away from this overbearing kid: your heart would beat faster, adrenaline would be released into the bloodstream, your pupils would dilate, sweat glands would be activated, and various other physiological changes would prepare you for the decision you made on how to deal with this anxiety-provoking situation.

The trigger to fight or flee – Whether you chose to fight or flee, the system would return to normal after the required physical exertion, and you would live to dread your next encounter with this aggravator. In medical school, the "bullies" or threats that you encounter may be more open to interpretation and less obviously identifiable: a demanding or unreasonable instructor, a seemingly unmanageable schedule, a financial crunch, a significant other delivering ultimatums, oversleeping and missing an exam, finding it impossible to grasp an important physiology concept, questioning whether you have the ability or desire to be a doctor, and so on. So while this response may be triggered by events you encounter—like having your car stolen with your award-winning lecture notes and textbooks inside it—it may also be generated by thoughts and attitudes that you hold about the event, like, "This will destroy any chance I have of passing this semester, lead to dismissal from medical school, and relegate me to selling cheap shoes at a flea market to earn a living."

The good news – The good news is that while you may not have control over events you encounter in medical school, such as the serious illness of a parent, you do have primary control over the thoughts and attitudes that you hold about those events and your interpretation and strategy development for dealing effectively with them. Making these thoughts and attitudes self-supporting rather than self-defeating will help tremendously with your success in medical school.

Learning to manage stress – In general, learning to manage stress is important for two reasons. First, the sensation of stress, the fight or flight response, is unpleasant at best, and frightening at its worst. It can range from the irritating uneasiness that prevents you from functioning at top form, to the panic attack that makes you wonder if you are having a heart attack, dying, or "going crazy." Second, if a stressor persists, it may impair the body's ability to cope, resulting in fatigue and illness.

The relatively new field of psychoneuroimmunology explores the relationship between psychological processes such as negative attitudes and negative emotions, the nervous and endocrine systems, and cells in the immune system. Such research studies why, for example, two medical students who are exposed to a flu virus will differ completely in their reaction to this exposure. One may be sick all winter, and the other may not so much as sneeze. Differences in thoughts and attitudes in general may be the variable that separates the successful copers from the unsuccessful copers in fighting off disease as well as keeping an optimistic view of one's environment. The ramifications of this particular example are self-evident when it comes to predicting which of these medical students will be more successful in meeting their goals. The successful medical student will be the one who masters the psychological attitudes and behavioral strategies that will enable the nervous and immune systems to function at their best.

What are the stressors of medical students? – The stress that you will inevitably feel falls within four domains:

1. The change in your self-concept as you make the transition from a medical school hopeful to an actual medical student.

2. The handling of your workload.

3. The demands you will place upon yourself.

4. The demands others will place upon you.

STRESSOR NUMBER ONE: Your self-concept is now changing – Self-concept is the image we have of ourselves. Our self-concept may be accurate, or inaccurate. It is highly subjective, affected by our family history, ongoing events, past and present interpersonal relationships, and our thoughts and attitudes. Our self-concept is also changeable. Obviously, a positive self-concept is desirable, and will give you the confidence to succeed and excel in medical school and life in general. Conversely, a negative self-concept will be an obstacle to feeling as powerful and positive as you need to feel to gain success.

You should be prepared for a shift in self-concept as you change from college graduate to entering medical student. Here's why. In high school and college you were "the cream of the crop," at the top in class rank. In medical school, however, you will be surrounded by peers of the same intellectual ability and achievement. And, while you may be the very student who graduates from medical school with the highest grades, it is also likely that you may find yourself in the middle range of your class in overall performance. This is a substantial change from what you are accustomed to, and if you do not expect this shift and explain it to yourself supportively, it can lead to a more negative self-concept. Here is how you can prevent this from happening:

1. Put things into their proper perspective – Remember that it is appropriate to feel some downward tuggings at your positive self-concept as you suddenly find yourself in the new situation of needing to work harder to achieve and excel the way you used to in high school and college. Don't let this throw you or worry you. Expect it. The medical school would not have accepted you if they were not confident that you are capable of performing to their standards.

2. View and treat other medical students as colleagues rather than as competitors – Competing with other medical students is self-defeating for several reasons.

First, there is no reason why all medical students can't excel; there is no grading curve, only consideration of individual performance. Second, in viewing others as competitors, you will be using an isolationist policy that will prevent you from enjoying the camaraderie of study groups, commiseration (remember, everyone's nervous about performance, no matter how blasé they may appear), and building relationships that may continue past medical school. It's entirely possible that you will meet an ideal partner for your future practice if you give yourself and other students the chance to develop in-depth relationships.

Finally, if your strategy is one of looking over your shoulder to stay ahead of the others, you will be adding the stress of a contest mentality to the already stressful rigors of academics. Medical school is not a competition; it is a time to get the best training you can, to perform to your optimal level, and to enjoy the pleasure of meeting and working with others who share your goals, trials, tribulations, and dreams.

3. Be proud of yourself – Don't compare yourself as a person and student to a "perfect person" (does anyone know one?), or to a "perfect student" (who doesn't know one?!). Instead, focus on your personal strengths and academic accomplishments. Perfectionists, many of whom are found in professional graduate programs, find this very difficult. They have the self-defeating habit of focusing on how far they fall from perfection. Rather, they need to revel in how far they exceed mediocrity. Use the theory of percentages to your advantage. What percentage of the population has achieved acceptance to medical school? What parent, friend, or relative wouldn't be proud to introduce you as a medical student? You are gifted, accomplished, and motivated. Remember this when you're tempted to scold yourself for not measuring up to your self-imposed expectation. Challenge yourself to create and live up to an appropriate standard of personhood and student performance. Go ahead and reward yourself for accomplishments. Resting on our laurels is a necessary practice at times. The "Yeah, I know I did well, but now I need to top that!" mentality will add counter-productive stress to your medical school experience.

STRESSOR NUMBER TWO: Handling your heavy workload – You will handle your workload successfully if you carefully follow these five recommendations.

1. Take care of yourself – First things first. You will handle your workload more successfully if you first handle the basic parts of your life successfully. This means eating well, sleeping well, not abusing substances of any kind (including caffeine, a fickle friend), exercising, making time for the positive people in your life, and regularly scheduling time for relaxation. If your body and mind are not in top form, the greatest study strategies and expenditures of time will not be as effective. Like a race car before a race, keep yourself in optimum shape physically and emotionally to endure the rigorous track.

2. Read this book and apply its strategies – Doing this will prepare you for the challenges ahead of you in such a way that you are preventive rather than reactive in dealing with the possible stumbling blocks to success. The study habits, strategies, and attitudes you will learn will be invaluable in giving yourself the best possible start in medical school.

3. Join or form a study group – Study groups provide a wealth of advantages. First, they provide accountability. When you are required to outline your particular assignment for use by the entire group, you must do so. It is human nature to come through for others more than we might come through for ourselves. Second, study groups make sense from an academic perspective. Dividing and conquering large masses of material, reviewing with others, and learning to prepare your assigned topics are all invaluable study strategies. Third, study groups are stress relievers. The camaraderie that comes from commiserating about and mastering difficult material is helpful not just from an academic perspective. It also provides a social outlet, enabling strong friendships to be formed as well as collegiality. Indeed, it may make for one of the most pleasurable aspects of your entire medical school experience.

4. Balance the various parts of your life – Another factor in handling your workload successfully rests in how well you balance your workload with the other parts of your life. Make no mistake: The rigors of medical school are all that you have heard but medical school must be carefully balanced and blended with the other areas of your life. Your role of medical student will consume most of your time, energy, and attention. However, you will also be expected to maintain other roles as well: daughter, son, fiancé, spouse, parent, sibling, relative, friend, hobbyist, committee member, ballplayer, and so on.

You must not dismiss these roles for a few reasons: First, the others in your life will not let you do so! Your parents will still expect you to call home, keep them posted, talk with your grandmother on her birthday, and so on. The same is true of significant others and good friends. Second, you will need these other roles and relationships to relax from the mental and physical exhaustion of your program of study. Remember, Ronald Reagan went horseback riding every Wednesday afternoon, no matter what was happening in the news. (Fill in a President of your choice—they have all had relaxation time scheduled or they would have been ineffective at their jobs).

Get away from it all – Remind yourself that "getting away from it all" can be a helpful technique if it results in a new sense of resilience, energy, and determination. You will need to believe this to give yourself permission to do so. Some ideas follow for quick "getaways" to help gain back study efficiency. Try to plan at least one per day. Many students find it easier to give themselves permission to "take a break" when they have already met some predetermined amount of study time. For example, you might spend Saturdays in the library from 9 AM to 5 PM seriously studying. At 5:01, tell yourself that the study part of your day is over, and that you need to renew yourself and to space your learning to be effective. Make plans with friends using this strategy, where you each hold the other accountable to show up at the library at 9 AM, and work conscientiously until 5 PM. Prearrange a short lunch with that friend to break up the day and to give yourself a chance to vent with a peer.

Quick "GETAWAY" ideas for stress management – Try the following ideas to help you relax and recharge:

1. Attend a movie that is upbeat, entertaining, and therefore not emotionally draining. The laughing it will evoke may help release endorphins to produce a natural high.

2. Exercise: run, jog, play softball, walk, do aerobics, do anything that will get your system going and release some endorphins for stress relief. Window shopping or serious shopping in a mall certainly qualifies as well.

3. Take both a quick nap and a hot shower (be sure to set an alarm clock before your nap). Some of our best ideas are born in the luxuriance of hot, soapy water.

4. Schedule a lunch or coffee with a student with whom you can commiserate. Swap coping strategies on how to manage the workload most effectively. Keep conversation upbeat.

5. Invest in a good relaxation audiotape. Any reputable bookstore will have a variety of them. This is a quick way to relieve stress and come away with a new feeling of centeredness.

6. Have a good joke book on hand and read two or three pages at a time as a study break. It helps to remember the humorous side of life whenever you become overly serious about the many life and death details of medicine.

7. Buy yourself a small treat: a box of Mallomars, a novel you've been wanting, wild new socks, or anything that brings you pleasure.

8. Listen to music. Have a wide range of selections on hand to best change your mood—from Beethoven to the Beach Boys, maybe even to Van Halen.

9. Clean your living space. The time away from studying will be well spent and give you a new sense of organization.

10. Take a ten minute mental vacation. Sit in a comfortable, quiet room. Close your eyes and slowly inhale deeply through your nose to the count of five. Hold your breath to the count of five. Now, exhale slowly through your mouth in such a way that you can hear yourself exhale. Next, envision yourself in a relaxing place where you would love to be—a favorite beach, vacation spot, cozy lodge, whatever scene brings you pleasure and relaxation. As you imagine the place, try to focus on the sensual aspects—sights, fragrances, tactile features, sounds, and tastes. If you have imagined a quiet beach, focus on the following: the comforting monotony of rolling waves, the tang of the sea air, the feel of the breeze on your arms, the cries of the sea gulls overhead, and the sweet nectar of summer's first watermelon or an ice-cold beer. Finally, repeat the deep breathing part of the exercise, this time thinking, "I am relaxed" as you exhale. Open your eyes slowly, and return to your schedule. (Note: If you want to be more scientific about the helpfulness of this exercise, rate your immediate stress level on a 1-low, 10-high scale prior to beginning the exercise. At its conclusion, give yourself a rating. If you see any decrease, particularly a significant one, you are an excellent candidate for relaxation audio-tapes available at any good bookstore.

11. Take another kind of mental vacation. Invest in a novel that takes you far away from the hassles of medical school. Reward yourself with chapter reading time in exchange for study time. Aim for mystery, adventure, or pure escapism as an easy way to "get away from it all" when reality won't allow it.

Relax regularly – Don't underestimate the value of using these exercises. Many medical students and residents minimize the need for a break and unfortunately utilize other self-defeating agents for battling stress quickly: caffeine, nicotine, alcohol to excess, and even drug abuse, prescription or nonprescription.

Watch out for coffee – Coffee is a great wake-up drink that is used by nearly everyone for a quick boost in alertness. It really works. But be careful, there is a connection between caffeine use and anxiety: Anxiety victims will react to the caffeine in one cup of coffee, or cola, or Mountain Dew as if it were four times that amount. This anxiety may build to a panic attack during times of stress, aided and abetted by caffeine ingestion. A good rule of thumb: If you tend to be more anxious than the average person, consider caffeine to be your enemy and switch to decaffeinated beverages. Nicotine, alcohol, and drugs can also have a negative impact on mood. Remember that as a doctor you will advocate natural stress management for your patients, rather than chemical agents. Follow your own advice and treat yourself as well as you will be telling your patients to treat themselves.

STRESSOR NUMBER THREE: The demands that you will place upon yourself – Three rigid beliefs you can demand of yourself will cause stress if you do not expect them and deal with them appropriately. They are:

1. "I must find the magic formula that makes medical school essentially stress-free."

2. "I must be at the top of my class and become a perfect doctor."

3. "There is no place for uncertainty in medical school or in the practice of medicine."

A truism – Remember: in medical school, you can be your own best advocate or your own worst enemy. It all depends upon how realistic your expectations of yourself are, and how you will talk yourself through the inevitable stress that you will experience.

The "magic formula" misconception – There is no magic formula. Expect medical school to be stressful. It is. But, you can manage the stress so that it doesn't become overwhelming and overshadow this very challenging and potentially enjoyable period of your life. Like the superwoman formula, the one that enables women to juggle job, marriage, and family effortlessly, it doesn't exist. (Believe me, I've searched for it!) Do your best to juggle your own priorities daily. The Time Management chapter of this book will assist with this. Keep in mind that medical school is your first priority for at least the next four years. You will need to learn your own special techniques for blending family, friends, and life maintenance so that your studies don't suffer, and neither do these other important areas of your life. This won't be easy. But consider it as an ongoing challenge and a continual reassessment of priorities for each day to make the best decisions and time allocations. If you observe a peer who seems to do particularly well at this juggling, ask how they do it! You may get some wonderful ideas or learn that you have a comrade in frustration—understand that either is desirable knowledge from a stress management viewpoint.

The "I must be perfect" misconception – As you begin medical school, the perfectionism that helped get you where you are today can work for you and against you. Your perfectionistic tendencies can work against you if you are so demanding of yourself that anxiety about performance replaces action in performance. For example, expect to find yourself scrutinizing the other medical students as your program of study begins. It is human to assign yourself a place in the "pecking order" of student performance. Don't be surprised if you feel that others seem to grasp course material more easily than you do, that they seem to have more free time than you do, and that the rigors of medical school seem less demanding for them than for you.

You could handle this unpleasant perception in one of two ways: one, in a best advocate way; the other, in a worst enemy way. In your worst enemy stance, you would ruminate about your feelings of inadequacy. Anxiety and inertia would replace action in dealing with the problem of assumed inferiority. In your best advocate stance, you would go the action route by doing the following: utilizing every possible study strategy to improve performance and confidence, joining or forming a study group to commiserate and cooperate in mastering material, and attempting to validate your observations about other students. In this case, you would gather your courage and share your perceptions of those seemingly "perfect students" you've been observing with those particular students. They will be flattered by your perception, and either acknowledge its validity or vehemently deny it.

Either way, you will be at an advantage. If they are feeling particularly confident about their performance, ask for pointers on their success. Most people love to be asked for input on areas in which they feel themselves to be expert. Such students may have a terrific study guide or study group to which they could direct you. If a seemingly perfect student states that appearances are deceiving and that he/she feels just as shaky as you do, you'll probably feel better knowing that you're not alone in your feelings of being "below the norm." Who knows, you may appear to be a "perfect student" to someone else. Confiding in others about the work load and how you're meeting your demands will go a long way in helping you deal with your workload realistically, and give you input on how others are doing as well.

Your goal is to put your studies first, to do the best you can do by utilizing every technique and resource available to you, and to enjoy the process at the same time. Statistically speaking, it is unlikely that you will be the top member of your class. Strive to be a very good member. It seems to me that the best doctors are composed of a unique combination of knowledge, judgement, compassion, and performance.

The "There can be no uncertainty in medicine" misconception – Of course there is! Medical school and your career in medicine will be fraught with uncertainty. Any field involving individual judgement calls will contain uncertainty. And you will experience uncertainty about medicine from your first day of class, if not before:

Do I have the "right stuff" to be a doctor?

Even if I have the "right stuff," do I want to be a doctor?

Am I able and/or willing to sacrifice what is required of a good doctor?

Did I make the right judgement call on that patient?

Should I ask for help with this situation?

. . . and so on.

These kinds of questions are not unique to medical students. They are asked by students in all kinds of professional programs: psychologists in training, dentistry students, veterinarian students, architects in training. Remember that uncertainty is natural and good. We should always feel free to analyze our decision making, and to feel comfortable to consult with others on our thoughts, feelings, and decisions. Medicine is scientific, but will always contain a human element, uncertainty.

When demands become too demanding – Stress manifests itself in three ways: physically, emotionally, and behaviorally. Physical symptoms can run the gamut from headache, difficulty swallowing, gain or loss in weight, chronic fatigue, and sexual difficulties. Emotional symptoms can range from irritability, racing thoughts, feelings of panic, episodes of crying, to withdrawal from others. Behaviorally, stress may manifest itself through increased smoking or drinking, high pitched nervous laughter, nail biting, teeth grinding, and so on. Since none of these symptoms are pleasant, several of them together may create a feeling of being overwhelmed.

When to seek help – If your feelings of stress are temporary and easily dispelled by taking a weekend off or venting to a supportive friend, fine. But, if you find the feeling of being overwhelmed continuing, it is a sign to get some help. Treat yourself as your own best advocate and ask, "Do you like the way you are feeling and performing?" (no) "Is this stress interfering with your ability to perform, resulting in greater stress?" (yes) "Doesn't it make sense to go to an expert in stress management to solve the problem?" (yes) "If such a person were available and you did not take advantage of them, wouldn't that be counter-productive?" (yes) While this may sound more like a Perry Mason cross-examination than self-advocacy, the point is the same: You must convince yourself that getting assistance is a tool for good problem solving. It shifts you from inaction to action, and is the first step in removing obstacles to feeling and performing better.

Where to seek help – Your medical school's Office of Student Affairs or Student Health Services are good first steps in seeking help. Think about it. Your school is equipped with counselors to help you deal with the stressors that are inevitable in medical school. Obviously if there is such a staff available, there is an expectation that students will need this service. Therefore, you should not feel sheepish or worried about seeking these services.

Another advantage of getting help from your school's counselors is that they will be experts in the issues germane to medical school and the resources that are available to help when you need direction. This may involve time off, financial aid, special consideration, input from helpful resources of which you were unaware, and so on. Remember, they have heard it all.

If you make the decision to seek help outside of the medical school community, choose a licensed or certified professional such as a psychologist, psychiatrist, or social worker. Referrals from respected friends are a good way to find a competent therapist. After that, go with your instincts. If you find yourself feeling more positive after a session, there is probably a good therapeutic match. If you leave a session feeling even more overwhelmed and confused than when you entered, or feel that your therapist is not on the same "wavelength" as you, try another for a better match. But do try. It makes no sense to feel worse when you can feel better.

STRESSOR NUMBER FOUR: The demands others will place upon you – Just when you've learned to adjust your self-concept and self-demands, you will now have to contend with the pressure of adjusting to the demands of the other people in your life—the medical faculty, family and friends, and patients.

The demands of the medical faculty – You will be perceived by the faculty as a student, but with more of a collegial feel in that relationship than you were used to in college. You will be seen as someone expected to put your medical studies first, and who should want to be both a medical expert and a compassionate provider to patients. They will expect you to be motivated to excel, and to overcome any obstacle to that goal. They will be demanding, but understanding of your situation if you communicate any special problem you may be facing. Remember that the faculty has experienced most of the challenges and frustrations of the medical school life. They have been in your position. Use the expertise of a trusted instructor when you want input on how to best cope with a particular aspect of medical school.

The demands of family and friends – Your family and friends can be obstacles to your success in medical school if they are not clear about the life-style required of a medical student. It is your challenge to be as direct and as tactful as possible about what your priorities are while in medical school. Quite simply, your first priority is to dedicate yourself completely to the study of medicine. While this does not equate with taking a vow of silence, it does mean that there will be significant changes in the way you interact with others. For example, you are no longer as available to others as you were before. You can't be. Your first commitment must be to yourself and your studies. You must make it clear to your family and friends that, while your behavior toward them may change (i.e., availability and frequency of contact), your feelings toward them are not involved in this change.

Supportive family and friends may not be happy about being on the back burner of your life, but they will understand. However, there might be some relationships in which you feel a constant battle over priorities, where you will find yourself feeling more frustrated than relaxed after contact. In these situations, you have a decision to make. If such people can't accept your judgement on how to best deal effectively with your medical studies, you may need to reconsider the relationship. With relatives, this may mean distancing yourself from these frustrating contacts if no amount of assertive discussion has resolved their demands. ("But why can't you just stop by your uncle's birthday party and <u>then</u> study for your exam?!") If a significant other is unwilling to accept your necessary life-style, you may need to evaluate if this person is the best match for you given the time-consuming career you have chosen.

Like the plant that thrives under the conditions of proper watering, sun, and temperature, you need to place yourself within those relationships and circumstances in which you thrive. Identify the people, activities, and attitudes that make you feel your best and most productive, and stick with them.

The demands of your patients – The perceptions patients you encounter will have of you will range from the flattering to the frustrating. Some will have both of those feelings. Your patients will see you as an expert, and despite a likely age difference, may look to you as a capable parent figure who will help them feel better. Being entrusted with this amount of control and power is heady, but it can also be frustrating. If your patients assume you are an expert, and place their lives in your hands, they are going to want positive results. Unfortunately, there will be times when you will not be able to help, despite your best intentions. The patient's ideal doctor is brilliant, compassionate, reliable, and personable. They want you to make them feel that they are important, that their health problems are important to you, and that you will cure them. Marcus Welby? Perhaps. Mostly, they want to feel that they are entrusting their lives to someone who will not betray them professionally or interpersonally.

Being the ideal doctor – You will need to develop a strategy to be as professional and personable as possible, while maintaining the distance that is required to prevent overinvolvement with patients. A common milestone to be overcome by both doctors and psychotherapists in training is that of taking your patients' problems home with you. This would impact negatively on your performance with all patients, not to mention your personal life. When you do find yourself feeling inadequate in helping to solve a patient's problem – cancer, for example – expect them to feel frustrated and even angry. And don't be surprised to experience these reactions from the previously adoring patient. It is all part of the doctor-patient relationship. Perhaps one of the best pieces of advice is the following: When dealing with patients, you don't have to help, you just have to try to help. Remember that when people are in pain or are frightened about their health, all kinds of emotional issues will emerge. You can be a help in this, a target in this, or a combination of both. Expect this scenario, consult with peers to relieve the stress, and just try to help.

In summary – You are now armed with some understanding of stress in medical school and a few strategies to deal with it. Being preventive in your approach, anticipating and preparing, will serve you best, and I hope that this chapter enables you to do so successfully. One last piece of advice: Have fun! Medical school, as with all challenges of this intensity, has the capacity to overwhelm you or exhilarate you. The attitude you take in approaching this chapter of your life will determine which emotional outcome will be yours.

Chapter 12

The Medical Specialties

Making your choice of a medical specialty – During your third and fourth years in medical school, you will decide what kind of doctor you wish to be. Throughout the fall of your fourth year, you will visit various residency programs in preparation for the Match. You will learn about the various specialties during your clinical clerkships from teachers, from your student affairs office, and from various books and pamphlets that are available. In addition, you will have the opportunity to take electives that will introduce you to different specialties, sometimes as early as the first year. Begin to think about your options now and take advantage of early opportunities to get exposure to the fields you are most attracted to. Your medical school's library and/or student affairs office has a large selection of such books or you may obtain them yourself. Below is a partial listing of information offered by various academies, societies, and foundations:

Plastic and Reconstructive Surgery, Plastic Surgery Education Foundation, 444 East Algonquin Rd., Arlington Hts., IL 60005, (708) 228-9900

Booklet of Information, American Board of Physical Medicine and Rehabilitation, Executive Director, 21 First Street, SW, Suite 674, Northwest Center, Rochester, MN 55902, (507) 282-1776

Careers in Preventive Medicine, American College of Preventive Medicine, 1015–15th St., NW, #403, Washington, DC 20005, (202) 789-0003

Directory of Graduate Medical Education Programs, American Medical Association, ATTN: Order Department, P.O. Box 109050, Chicago, IL 60610, (800) 621-8335, ($48.00 + s/h and tax)

Neurologist Brochure, American Academy of Neurology, 2221 University Avenue, SE, Suite 335, Minneapolis, MN 55414, (612) 623-8115

Selected Career Paths in Medicine, American College of Physicians, 6th Street at Race, Philadelphia, PA 19106, (800) 523-1546

What is Exercise Physiology? American College of Sports Medicine Today, and *The Sports Medicine Umbrella,* American College of Sports Medicine, Public Information Department, P.O. Box 1440, Indianapolis, IN 46206-1440, (317) 637-9200

Your Career in Pediatrics, American Academy of Pediatrics, 141 Northwest Point Blvd., Elk Grove Village, IL 60007, (800) 433-9016

Description of recognized specialties – The following are descriptions of the various specialties of medicine. This material is modified from:

Which Medical Specialist For You, The American Board of Medical Specialties, 1007 Church Street, Suite 404, Evanston, IL 60201-5913, Telephone (708) 491-9091.

For a more complete description of each medical specialty write to the American Board of Medical Specialties for a copy of their booklet.

Allergy and Immunology – An allergist-immunologist is a certified internist or pediatrician expert in the evaluation, physical and laboratory diagnosis, and management of disorders potentially involving the immune system. Selected experts may receive special certification in "Diagnostic Laboratory Immunology" after additional training in the various laboratory procedures required to analyze both the function and malfunction of the immune system. Dual certification programs are now available at some training centers for preparation of candidates with expertise in allergy-immunology and adult rheumatology and allergy-immunology and pediatric pulmonology.

Anesthesiology – The anesthesiologist is a physician who, following medical school graduation and at least four years of postgraduate training, has the principal task of providing pain relief and maintenance, or restoration, of a stable condition during and immediately following an operation, or an obstetric or diagnostic procedure. The anesthesiologist assesses the risk of the patient undergoing surgery and optimizes the patient's condition prior to, during, and after surgery. Anesthesiologists diagnose and treat acute and long-standing pain problems and treat patients who have critical illnesses or are severely injured. Anesthesiologists direct resuscitation in cardiac or respiratory emergencies including the provision of artificial ventilation.

Critical Care Medicine – The anesthesiologist who specializes in critical care medicine must receive additional training because the requisite knowledge and skills extend beyond anesthesiology training and cross traditional specialty lines. Anesthesiologists trained in critical-care are qualified to diagnose, treat, and support patients with multiple organ dysfunction. They may have administrative responsibilities for intensive-care units and may participate in the training and medical direction of essential health care professionals such as nurses, respiratory therapists, and physicians in training. The primary work place is an intensive- or critical-care unit.

Pain Management – The anesthesiologist who specializes in pain management also must receive additional training to treat patients within the entire range of painful disorders with knowledge required for the diagnosis and management of patients with pain.

Colon and Rectal Surgery – A board certified colon and rectal surgeon has completed at least five years of residency training in general surgery and one additional year devoted entirely to colon and rectal surgery. He/she has then passed both the written (Qualifying) and oral (Certifying) examinations given by the American Board of Colon and Rectal Surgery. As a result of their training and experience, colon and rectal surgeons are able to diagnose and treat various diseases of the intestinal tract, colon, rectum, anal canal, and perianal area by medical and surgical means. They are also able to deal surgically with other organs and tissues (such as the liver, urinary, and female reproductive system) involved with primary intestinal disease. A colon and rectal surgeon has expertise to diagnose and often manage anorectal conditions such as hemorrhoids, fissures, abscesses, and fistulae. Colon and rectal surgeons also perform endoscopic procedures to detect and treat conditions of the bowel lining. Colon and rectal surgeons perform abdominal surgical procedures involving the small bowel, colon, and rectum. These include treatment of inflammatory bowel diseases as well as diverticulitis and cancer.

Dermatology – A dermatologist is a physician who has expertise in the diagnosis, and treatment of pediatric and adult patients with benign and malignant disorders of the skin, mouth, external genitalia, hair and nails, as well as a number of sexually transmitted diseases. The dermatologist also has expertise in the management of cosmetic disorders of the skin such as hair loss and scars. To be certified as a dermatologist, a physician must have had at least four years of residency training. The first broad-based, general clinical year is followed by three years of intensive training in dermatology including dermatopathology and dermatologic surgery. In addition to the successful completion of the four years of required training, the certification process includes a comprehensive examination administered by the American Board of Dermatology. A dermatologist may subspecialize and become certified for special qualification as follows:

Dermatopathology – Special qualification in dermatopathology, signifying advanced competence, can be obtained by either a board certified dermatologist or a pathologist. Special qualification involves further extensive training and experience in the evaluation of tissue specimens submitted from dermatologic patients. These evaluations include the examination and interpretation of microscopic slides of thin tissue sections and smears, and scrapings from lesions of skin.

Immunodermatology – An immunodermatologist, through additional special training, has developed expertise in the study of the cause, diagnosis, treatment, and outcome of skin diseases involving the immune system. These physicians have a basic understanding of such diseases from the perspective of anatomic and clinical pathology, along with the accurate interpretation of immunologic analyses of tissue cells and body fluids. The immunodermatologist is knowledgeable and experienced in utilizing many forms of immunological treatments.

Emergency Medicine – Emergency medicine is the medical specialty that focuses on the immediate decision making and action necessary to prevent death or any further disability. It is primarily hospital emergency department-based, but with extensive prehospital responsibilities for emergency medical systems. The emergency physician provides immediate initial recognition, evaluation, care, and disposition of a generally undifferentiated population of patients in response to acute illness and injury.

Pediatric Emergency Medicine – The pediatric emergency physician is trained to manage emergencies in infants and children.

Sports Medicine – The emergency medicine physician specializing in sports medicine is trained to be responsible for not only the enhancement of health and fitness but also the prevention of injury and illness. Knowledge about exercise physiology, biomechanics, nutrition, psychology, physical rehabilitation, and epidemiology are essential.

Medical Toxicology – Physicians certified in emergency medicine and in different areas of primary-care medicine who are certified in medical toxicology have special knowledge about the evaluation and management of patients with accidental or intentional poisoning through exposure to prescription and non-prescription medications, drugs of abuse, household or industrial toxins, and environmental toxins. These physicians provide specialty consultations through affiliations with regional poison control centers, or are recognized as specialists and provide toxicological consultations within their respective institutions.

Family practice – Family physicians are trained to prevent, diagnose, and treat a wide variety of ailments in patients of all ages. They have received a broad range of training that includes surgery, psychiatry, internal medicine, obstetrics and gynecology, pediatrics, and geriatrics. They place special emphasis on care of families on a continuing basis utilizing consultations and community resources when appropriate. They are able to apply modern techniques to prevention, diagnosis, and treatment of the vast majority of common illnesses and injuries.

Geriatric Medicine – With additional training, a family physician can become certified in geriatrics. A family physician with an added certificate in geriatrics is capable of advising older patients in the prevention, diagnosis, treatment, and rehabilitation of disorders common to old age.

Sports Medicine – The family physician specializing in sports medicine is trained to be responsible for continuous care in the field of sports medicine, not only the enhancement of health and fitness but the prevention of injury and illness.

Internal Medicine – The general internist is a personal physician who provides long-term, comprehensive care in the office and the hospital, managing both common illnesses and complex problems for adolescents, adults, and the elderly. General internists are trained in the essentials of primary-care internal medicine, which incorporates an understanding of disease prevention, wellness, substance abuse, mental health, and effective treatment of common problems of the eyes, ears, skin, nervous system, and reproductive organs. All internists are trained in the subspecialty areas of emergency internal medicine and critical care.

Adolescent Medicine – The general internist specializing in adolescent medicine concentrates on the unique health care needs of adolescents in special circumstances and coordinates the subspecialty care required for youth, as well as the planning and supervision for transitional health care services to adult health care.

Cardiovascular Medicine – Cardiologists subspecialize in diseases of the heart, lungs, and blood vessels and manage cardiac conditions such as heart attacks and abnormal heart beat rhythms.

Clinical Cardiac Electrophysiology – This is a field of narrow interest within the subspecialty of cardiology. Cardiac Electrophysiology involves complicated technical procedures to evaluate heart rhythms and determine appropriate treatment. These procedures are performed in a variety of settings including emergency and operating rooms, and intensive-care units.

Critical Care Medicine – The internist critical-care specialist manages life-threatening disorders in intensive-care units and other hospital settings. Shock, coma, heart failure, trauma, respiratory arrest, drug overdoses, massive bleeding, and kidney failure are examples of conditions requiring critical care by internists.

Diagnostic Laboratory Immunology – This is a subspecialty field in which laboratory tests and complex procedures are used to diagnose and treat disorders characterized by defective responses of the immune systems.

Endocrinology – The endocrinologist concentrates on disorders of the endocrine glands. Endocrinology also deals with disorders such as diabetes, metabolic and nutritional disorders, pituitary diseases, and menstrual and sexual problems.

Gastroenterology – The subspecialty of the digestive organs involves the stomach, bowels, liver, and gallbladder. The gastroenterologist treats conditions such as abdominal pain, ulcers, diarrhea, cancer, and jaundice. Gastroenterologists perform complex diagnostic and therapeutic procedures using lighted scopes to see internal organs. They consult with surgeons when abdominal operations are indicated.

Geriatric Medicine – The internist certified in geriatric medicine has special knowledge of the aging process and special skills in the diagnostic, therapeutic, preventive, and rehabilitative aspects of illness in the elderly. Geriatricians are trained to recognize the unusual presentations of illness and drug interactions, to utilize resources such as community social services, and to assist with special ethical issues in the care of the elderly. Examples of common geriatric conditions include incontinence, falls, Parkinson's disease, Alzheimer's disease, and other dementias.

Hematology – Hematologists subspecialize in diseases of the blood, spleen, and lymph glands. They treat conditions such as anemia, clotting disorders, sickle cell disease, hemophilia, leukemia, and lymphoma. They perform transfusions and biopsy the bone marrow for analysis.

Infectious Diseases – These subspecialists deal with infectious diseases of all types and in all organs. Conditions requiring selective use of antibiotics call for this special skill.

Medical Oncology – The medical oncologist specializes in the diagnosis and treatment of cancer and benign and malignant tumors. These subspecialists decide on and administer chemotherapy for malignancy as well as consult with surgeons and radiotherapists on other treatments for cancer.

Nephrology – The nephrologist is concerned with disorders of the kidney, high blood pressure, fluid and mineral balance, dialysis of body wastes when the kidneys do not function, and consultation with surgeons about kidney transplantation.

Pulmonary Diseases – Pulmonary disease is the subspecialty concerned with diseases of the lungs and airways. Pulmonologists test lung functions, endoscope the bronchial airways and prescribe and monitor mechanical assistance to ventilation. Many pulmonary disease experts are also expert in critical care.

Rheumatology – The rheumatologist is concerned with diseases of joints, muscle, bones, and tendons. He diagnoses and treats arthritis, back pain, muscle strains, common athletic injuries, and "collagen" diseases.

Sports Medicine – The physician specializing in sports medicine is trained to be responsible for continuous care in the field of sports medicine, not only the enhancement of health and fitness but the prevention of injury and illness. The sports medicine physician requires special education to provide the knowledge to improve the health care of the individual engaged in physical exercise (sports) whether as an individual or in team participation.

Allergy and Immunology – The subspecialty of allergy and immunology is represented by a conjoint board of the American Board of Internal Medicine and the American Board of Pediatrics, called the American Board of Allergy and Immunology.

Medical Genetics – The medical geneticist is a specialist trained in the diagnostic and therapeutic procedures for patients with genetic-linked diseases. Individual genetic diseases can now be recognized by suitably trained specialists with the assistance of modern cytogenetic, radiologic, and biochemical testing. Such diagnostic information can assist the medical geneticist in genetic counseling, the implementation of needed therapeutic interventions, and prospective prevention through prenatal diagnosis.

Neurological Surgery – Neurological surgery is the discipline of medicine and that specialty of surgery which provides the operative and non-operative management (i.e., prevention, diagnosis, treatment, critical-care, and rehabilitation) of disorders of the nervous system, and management of pain.

Critical-Care Medicine – The neurological surgeon who has received additional training in critical-care medicine is a specialist whose knowledge involves all aspects of management of the critically ill patient in the intensive-care unit (ICU).

Neurology – The speciality of neurology is concerned with the diagnosis and treatment of all categories of disease or impaired function of the brain, spinal cord, peripheral nerves, muscles, and autonomic nervous system, as well as the blood vessels that relate to these structures. The neurologist serves as a consultant to other physicians but is often the primary physician and may render all levels of care commensurate with his training. Formal subspecialization is available for added qualification in clinical neurophysiology, involving one additional year of training in the diagnosis and management of nervous system disorders using electrophysiological techniques.

Nuclear Medicine – Nuclear medicine is the medical specialty that employs the nuclear properties of radioactive and stable nuclides in diagnosis, therapy, and research. These properties are used to evaluate metabolic, physiologic, and pathologic conditions in both the clinical and laboratory setting. A specialist in nuclear medicine has been awarded a medical degree, has satisfactorily completed two or more years of residency training in a general medical specialty, two additional years of nuclear medicine residency, and has passed a written examination. The professional competence of nuclear medicine physicians is in the diagnostic and therapeutic uses of radionuclides including: radioimmunoassay; therapy with radioisotopically labelled antibodies; positron emission tomography (PET); and single-proton emission computerized tomography (SPECT). Additionally, the nuclear medicine physician has special knowledge in the biologic effects of radiation exposure; the principles of radiation safety and protection; the management of patients who have been exposed to ionizing radiation; and special knowledge in the physical sciences encompassing the fundamentals of nuclear physics and nuclear magnetic resonance; the principles and operation of radiation detection and nuclear imaging instrumentation systems; statistics and fundamentals of computer sciences. The nuclear medicine specialist serves as a consultant to physicians, obtaining pertinent information from patients as necessary by means of history and physical examination and selecting and carrying out diagnostic or therapeutic uses of radionuclides.

Obstetrics and Gynecology – Obstetrician/gynecologists are physicians who, by virtue of satisfactory completion of a defined course of graduate medical education and appropriate certification, possess special knowledge, skills, and professional capability in the medical and surgical care of the female reproductive system and associated disorders.

Critical-Care Medicine – The obstetrician/gynecologist who has additional training in critical-care medicine is a specialist in all aspects of management of the critically ill patient and whose base of operation is the intensive-care unit (ICU).

Gynecologic Oncology – A gynecologic oncologist is trained to provide consultation and comprehensive management of patients with gynecologic cancer and whose activity includes the practice of gynecologic oncology in an institutional setting with all the effective forms of cancer therapy.

Maternal-Fetal Medicine – A maternal-fetal medicine specialist is prepared to care for or provide consultation on patients with complications of pregnancy. This requires advanced knowledge in the obstetrical, medical, and surgical complications of pregnancy and their effect on both the mother and the fetus.

Reproductive Endocrinology – A reproductive endocrinologist is a specialist capable of managing complex problems relating to reproductive endocrinology and infertility.

Ophthalmology – An ophthalmologist has had at least one year of general medical postgraduate training and has subsequently completed three or more additional years of postgraduate medical and surgical training in an ophthalmology training program. Ophthalmologists are trained to diagnose, monitor, and medically or surgically treat all eyelid and orbital problems affecting the eye and visual pathways and to diagnose, monitor, and treat all eye and visual disorders.

Orthopaedic Surgery – Orthopaedic surgery is the medical specialty that includes the preservation, investigation, and restoration of the form and function of the extremities, spine, and associated structures by medical, surgical, and physical means. Congenital deformities, trauma, infections, tumors, and metabolic disturbances of the musculoskeletal system are problems cared for by the orthopaedic surgeon.

Hand Surgery – Hand surgery is that special field of medicine that includes the investigation, preservation, and restoration by medical, surgical, and rehabilitative means of all structures of the upper extremity directly affecting the form and function of the hand and wrist.

Otolaryngology – An otolaryngologist/head and neck surgeon is a physician who has been prepared by accredited residency programs to provide comprehensive medical and surgical care of patients with diseases and disorders that affect the ears, the respiratory and upper alimentary systems, and the related structures. The required five years of postgraduate training includes one or more years of general surgery and three or more years of otolaryngology.

Otology/Neurotology – The otolaryngologist and head and neck surgeon who specializes in otology/neurotology must receive training in the diagnosis, management, prevention, cure, and care of patients with diseases of the ear and temporal bone including disorders of hearing and balance.

Pediatric Otolaryngology – The pediatric otolaryngologist has special expertise in the management of infants and children with disorders that include congenital and acquired conditions involving the aerodigestive tract, nose and paranasal sinuses, the ear, and other areas of the head and neck.

Pathology – Pathology is that specialty dealing with the causes and nature of disease. A certified specialist in pathology completed an approved postgraduate program in pathology and an evaluation process, including an examination administered by The American Board of Pathology. Pathologists use their skills and knowledge for the diagnosis, exclusion, and monitoring of disease through information gathered from the microscopic examination of tissue specimens, cells, and body fluids, and from clinical laboratory tests on body fluids and secretions. A certified specialist in pathology may subspecialize and become certified in one of the following areas:

Blood Banking – A physician specializing in blood banking is responsible for the maintenance of an adequate blood supply, donor and recipient safety, and appropriate blood utilization.

Chemical Pathology – A chemical pathologist is expert in biochemistry and is concerned with the application of biochemical data to the detection, confirmation, or monitoring of disease.

Cytopathology – A cytopathologist is a certified anatomic pathologist who, in addition, has had special training and experience in the diagnosis of human disease by means of the study of cells.

Dermatopathology – A dermatopathologist is expert in diagnosing and monitoring disease of the skin including infectious immunologic, degenerative, and neoplastic diseases.

Forensic Pathology – A forensic pathologist is expert in investigating and evaluating cases of sudden, unexpected, suspicious, and violent death as well as other classes of death defined by law.

Hematology – A hematologist/pathologist is expert in diseases that affect blood cells, blood clotting mechanisms, bone marrow, skills essential for the laboratory diagnosis of anemias, leukemias, lymphomas, and bleeding and blood clotting disorders.

Immunopathology – An immunopathologist is concerned with the scientific study of the causes, diagnosis, and prognosis of disease by the application of immunological principles to the analysis of tissues, cells, and body fluids.

Medical Microbiology – A medical microbiologist has expertise in the isolation and identification of microbes that cause disease.

Neuropathology – A neuropathologist is expert in the diagnosis of disease of the nervous system and skeletal muscles and functions as a consultant primarily to neurologists and neurosurgeons.

Pediatric Pathology – The specialist in pediatric pathology is an expert in the laboratory diagnosis of diseases that occur during fetal growth and infant and childhood development.

Pediatrics – Pediatrics is the specialty concerned with the physical, emotional, and social health of children from birth to young adulthood. Pediatric care ranges from preventive health care to the diagnosis and treatment of acute and chronic diseases. Pediatrics also deals with biological, social, and environmental influences on the developing child and with the impact of disease on development. A pediatrician may subspecialize in:

Adolescent Medicine – The pediatrician specializing in adolescent medicine is a multidisciplinary health care specialist trained in the unique physical, psychological, and social characteristics of adolescents, their health care problems and needs.

Medical Toxicology – A pediatric medical toxicologist is a physician with specialized training that focuses on the evaluation and management of patients with accidental or intentional poisoning through exposure to prescription and non-prescription medications, drugs of abuse, household or industrial toxins, and environmental toxins.

Neonatal-Perinatal Medicine – A specialist in neonatal-perinatal medicine is the principal care provider for sick newborn infants.

Pediatric Cardiologist – A pediatric cardiologist is a specialist for children from fetal life to young adulthood who provides comprehensive care to patients with cardiovascular problems.

Pediatric Critical-Care Medicine – This specialist has competence in advanced life support for children from the neonate to the adolescent.

Pediatric Endocrinologist – A pediatric endocrinologist provides expert care to infants, children, and adolescents who have diseases that result from an abnormality in the endocrine glands including diabetes mellitus, growth failure, unusual size for age, early or late pubertal development, birth defects, etc.

Pediatric Emergency Medicine – The pediatric emergency physician is one who has special qualifications to manage emergencies in children.

Pediatric Gastroenterology – A pediatric gastroenterologist has competence in the clinical diagnosis and medical treatment of disorders of the digestive system of children and adolescents.

Pediatric Hematologist-Oncologist – A pediatric hematologist-oncologist is a specialized physician trained in the recognition and management of hematologic (blood disorders) and oncologic (cancerous) diseases in infants, children, and adolescents.

Pediatric Infectious Disease – The pediatric infectious disease subspecialist is a physician who cares for children in the treatment and prevention of infectious diseases.

Pediatric Nephrologist – A pediatric nephrologist is a medical specialist for children from fetal life to young adulthood who deals with the normal and abnormal development and maturation of the kidney and the urinary tract, the mechanisms by which the kidney can be damaged, the evaluation and treatment of renal diseases, fluid and electrolyte abnormalities, hypertension, and renal replacement therapy.

Pediatric Pulmonologist – The pediatric pulmonologist is dedicated to the prevention and treatment of all respiratory diseases affecting infants, children and young adults.

Pediatric Rheumatology – A pediatric rheumatology subspecialist is a pediatrician whose primary responsibilities are to treat and provide an excellent level of patient care for the infant, child, or adolescent with a rheumatic or related disease.

Pediatric Sports Medicine – A pediatric sports medicine subspecialist is a pediatrician with special training and education in the body of knowledge and the broad area of health care involving exercise as an essential component of health throughout life, medical supervision of recreational and competitive athletes and all those who exercise, and exercise for prevention and treatment of disease and injury.

Physical Medicine and Rehabilitation – Physical medicine and rehabilitation, also referred to as rehabilitation medicine, is the medical specialty concerned with diagnosing, evaluating, and treating patients with impairments and/or disabilities that involve musculoskeletal, neurologic, cardiovascular, or other body systems. The primary focus is on maximal restoration of physical, psychological, social and vocational function, and on alleviation of pain. For diagnosis and evaluation, a physiatrist may include the techniques of electromyography and electrodiagnosis as supplements to the standard history, physical, x-ray, and laboratory exams. In addition to traditional treatment modes, this specialist may use therapeutic exercise, prosthetics, orthotics, and mechanical and electrical devices.

Plastic Surgery – The specialty of plastic surgery deals with the repair and reconstruction of defects of form and function of the integument and its underlying musculoskeletal system, with emphasis on the craniofacial structures, the oropharynx, the upper and lower limbs, the breast, and the external genitalia. It includes aesthetic surgery of structures with undesirable form. Special knowledge and skill in the design and transfer of flaps, in the transplantation of tissues, and in the replantation of structures are vital to these ends, as is skill in excisional surgery, in management of complex wounds, and in the use of alloplastic materials. Knowledge of surgical design, surgical diagnosis, surgical and artistic anatomy, surgical pathology, surgical oncology, surgical physiology and pharmacology and bacteriology, biomechanics, embryology, and surgical instrumentation are fundamental to this specialty. The judgment and technical capability for achieving satisfactory surgical results are mandatory qualities for the plastic surgeon. The minimum commitment in years of training is five with most individuals training for seven years. A certified specialist in plastic surgery may subspecialize and be certified for special qualifications in surgery of the hand.

Preventive Medicine – Preventive medicine is that specialty that focuses on the health of individuals and defined populations in order to protect, promote and maintain health and well-being, and to prevent disease, disability and premature death. In addition to the knowledge of basic and clinical sciences and the skills common to all physicians, the distinctive components of preventive medicine include: biostatistics, epidemiology, health services administration, environmental and occupational influences on health, social and behavioral influences on health, and measures that prevent the occurrence, progression, and disabling effects of disease or injury.

  Medical Toxicology – The specialty of preventive medicine also provides for the opportunity of subspecialty training in medical toxicology with a focus on the evaluation and management of patients with accidental or intentional poisoning through exposure to prescription and non-prescription medications, drugs of abuse, household or industrial toxins, and harmful environmental toxins.

Psychiatry – A psychiatrist is a physician who specializes in the prevention, diagnosis, and treatment of mental, addictive and emotional disorders (e.g., psychoses, depression, anxiety disorders, substance abuse disorders, developmental disabilities, sexual dysfunctions, adjustment reactions.) The psychiatrist has had four years of specialized training after obtaining a medical degree. He or she is thus able to understand the biological, psychological, and social components of illness and is qualified to order diagnostic laboratory tests and to prescribe medications, as well as to evaluate and treat psychological and interpersonal problems. The psychiatrist is also prepared to intervene with individuals and families who are coping with stress, crises, and other problems in living. Some psychiatrists have also had further training in the following specialized areas:

Addiction Psychiatry – One additional year of training qualifies a psychiatrist in the understanding of addictive disorders and the special and emotional problems that are related to addiction and substance abuse.

Child and Adolescent Psychiatry – A child and adolescent psychiatrist has two additional years of training in the diagnosis and treatment of psychiatric disorders of childhood and adolescence.

Clinical Neurophysiology – This subspecialty involves one additional year of training in the diagnosis and management of nervous system disorders using electrophysiological techniques.

Forensic Psychiatry – The field of forensic psychiatry is also available for subspecialization and requires special skills in knowledge and evaluation of certain diagnostic groups of patients that include: sexual disorders, antisocial personality disorders, paranoid disorders, and addictive disorders. The forensic psychiatrist requires special skills and training to perform careful observations for malingering, the utilization of ancillary information such as police reports, interviews with relatives and witnesses, and review of medical records.

Geriatric Psychiatry – A geriatric psychiatrist has devoted one additional year of training to the diagnosis and treatment of mental, addictive, and emotional disorders of the elderly.

Radiology – Radiologists use various forms of radiant energy to detect and manage disease and injuries. The several branches of radiology are:

Diagnostic Radiological Physics – Diagnostic radiological physics deals with the diagnostic applications of roentgen rays, gamma rays from sealed sources, ultrasonic radiation, radio-frequency radiation, and the equipment associated with their production and use.

Diagnostic Radiology – This branch of radiology utilizes all modalities of radiant energy in medical diagnoses and therapeutic procedures needing radiologic guidance. This includes, but is not restricted to, imaging techniques and methodologies utilizing radiations emitted by x-ray tubes, radionuclides, and ultrasonographic devices.

Medical Nuclear Physics – Medical nuclear physics deals with (1) the therapeutic and diagnostic application of radionuclides (except those used in sealed sources for therapeutic purposes), and (2) the equipment associated with their production and use.

Nuclear Radiology – Nuclear radiology involves the analysis and imaging of radionuclides and radiolabeled substances in vitro and in vivo for diagnosis and the administration of radionuclides and radiolabeled substances for the treatment of disease.

Radiological Physics – This branch of medical physics includes therapeutic radiological physics, diagnostic radiological physics, and medical nuclear physics; including radiation safety.

Therapeutic Radiological Physics – This branch of medical physics deals with (1) the therapeutic applications of roentgen rays, of gamma rays, of electron and other charged particle beams, of neutrons, and of radiations from sealed radionuclide sources, and (2) the equipment associated with their production and use.

Therapeutic Radiology – Therapeutic radiology (radiation oncology) is that branch of radiology that deals with the therapeutic application of radiant energy and its modifiers and the study and management of disease, especially malignant tumors.

General Surgery – A general surgeon is a specialist prepared to manage a broad spectrum of surgical conditions affecting almost any area of the body. The surgeon makes the diagnoses and provides the preoperative, operative, and postoperative care to surgical patients and is usually responsible for the comprehensive management of the trauma victim and the critically ill. During at least a five-year educational period after obtaining a medical degree, the surgeon acquires knowledge and technical skills in congenital, infectious, metabolic, and neoplastic problems relating to the head and neck, breast, abdomen, extremities including the hand, and the gastrointestinal, vascular, and endocrine systems. The surgeon uses a variety of diagnostic techniques, including endoscopy, for observing internal structures, and may use specialized instruments during operative procedures. A general surgeon is expected to be familiar with the salient features of other surgical specialties in order to recognize problems in those areas and to know when to refer a patient to another specialist. Other areas of special expertise are recognized within the discipline of general surgery, requiring additional training and further examination.

General Vascular Surgery – This is a surgeon with special qualifications in the management of surgical disorders of the blood vessels excluding those immediately adjacent to the heart, lungs, or brain.

Pediatric Surgery – This surgeon has special qualifications in the management of surgical conditions in premature and newborn infants, children, and adolescents.

Surgical Critical-Care – Critical-care surgeons have special qualifications in the management of the critically ill and postoperative patient, particularly the trauma victim, in the emergency room, intensive care unit, trauma unit, and other similar settings.

Surgery of the Hand – A surgeon with special qualifications in the management of surgical disorders of the hand.

Thoracic Surgery – Thoracic surgery encompasses the operative, peri-operative, and critical care of patients with pathologic conditions within the chest. Included is the surgical care of coronary artery disease, lung cancers, abnormalities of the great vessels and heart valves, congenital anomalies, tumors of the mediastinum, and diseases of the diaphragm. The management of the airway and injuries of the chest is within the scope of the specialty. Certification by the American Board of Thoracic Surgery requires previous certification by the American Board of Surgery, plus a minimum two-year period of training in thoracic surgery, as well as passage of a two-part examination. Thoracic surgeons have substantial knowledge of cardio-respiratory physiology and oncology, as well as capability in the use of extracorporeal circulation, cardiac assist devices, management of dysrhythmias, pleural drainage, respiratory support systems, endoscopy, and invasive and non-invasive diagnostic techniques.

Urology – A specialist in urology is certified by the American Board of Urology to manage benign and malignant medical and surgical disorders of the adrenal gland and of the genitourinary system. Urologists have comprehensive knowledge of, and skills in, endoscopic, percutaneous, and open surgery of congenital and acquired conditions of the reproductive and urinary systems and their contiguous structures.

Chapter 13

Medical Ethics
by Rosamond Rhodes, Ph.D.

The Mount Sinai School of Medicine

Introduction – Medical ethics is a critically important part of a physician's education. Decisions made daily in the medical setting have dramatic health consequences for the patient. Such decisions are made based on medical facts and medical science, but they must also reflect moral deliberation. Consider the following three arguments:

> **Argument (1)** Whenever a person acts, the action performed could be either right or wrong.

> **Argument (2)** Whenever a person chooses an action, a different choice might have been better or worse.

> **Argument (3)** The long-range consequences of an action might have been more or less favorable than the consequences of the alternatives.

These three arguments imply that every action is part of the moral domain and that all actions are subject to moral evaluation.

Ethics can be discussed from the perspective of virtue, utility, principles, or rights. Since most contemporary discussion of medical ethics focuses on the patient's rights, the obligations of physicians, and the right to health care, rights theory will be the framework for this chapter. And because feelings play an important role in right action, we must also consider the emotions of physicians. Our goal is not to offer a detailed outline of ethical theory but rather to provide enough general background to illustrate the moral complexity of common encounters in medical practice.

Feelings – Ethical behavior includes both a theoretical analysis and an emotional component as necessary features of virtuous human interaction. If you act solely from the warm feelings of goodwill, without attending to principles such as justice, you will miss the mark. The same is true when acting solely from principles, without the feelings of goodwill. Virtuous people are morally excellent because they have principles and extend goodwill to everyone they meet. They 'see' the situation accurately because they are not swayed by inappropriate feelings and they understand what has to be done. They are likely to do the right thing because they love their fellow man. Caring feelings, along with attention to principles and theoretical analysis, are the basic requirements of morality.

The doctor/patient relationship – Between a doctor and her patient, there are inequalities in medical knowledge, in physical well-being, and in fear. These inequalities give the physician/patient relationship its own special character. The good doctor will not look to her own interests, but, rather, to those of her patients, caring for them to promote their well-being. The good doctor will feel goodwill toward her patients, and from that feeling she will be able to give each patient what is morally due.

Sometimes patients who are given good medical treatment become upset or angry if they feel that their doctor does not care about them personally. From the perspective of principles alone, this is a peculiar response since the physician has fulfilled her obligation. But more is required of the physician. The patient correctly perceives a lack of doctorly love as inappropriate because the good doctor should love her patients.

The need for caring in the doctor/patient relationship also explains why physicians find it difficult to fulfill their obligations to the non-compliant or hateful patient. The lack of love makes it hard to do one's duty; only the commitment to principles enables the physician to overcome her disinclination to give proper treatment. On the other hand, an excess amount of love and concern for a patient may lead the physician to be unjust and give her patient more than what is due. Excessive caring may incline a physician to break protocol and administer a different drug or to provide a second or third or fourth transplant organ to a beloved patient who, according to standards of just distribution, would otherwise be denied retransplantation. A virtuous doctor would recognize what morality required and, with goodwill, do the right thing.

Rights and duties – According to rights theory, whenever someone has a right, someone else has a duty. The relationship of rights and duties can be seen as the two sides of a coin; one part of the relationship does not exist without the other. For example, if a patient has an appointment with her physician at 2:00 PM, the patient has the right to have her physician available at 2:00 PM, and the physician has the duty to be available at that time. In rights/duties relationships, individuals typically have reciprocal rights and duties to each other. Thus, the patient also has the duty to keep the appointment, and her physician has the right to expect her to keep it.

This reciprocity is often the model for moral relationships. In the doctor/patient relationship, as in the parent/child relationship however, reciprocity remains an open question. For example, while parental duties create many rights for children (food, clothing, shelter, education, nurturing), and parents may wish to assign duties (chores) to their children, a child's failure to complete those chores would not abrogate the persisting parental duties. Similarly, a patient's failure to meet an obligation by coming late, missing appointments, or noncompliance, does not cancel the physician's duty to treat.

General duties – There are some duties that everyone has. From the correlation of rights and duties, this would suggest that everyone has the corresponding rights.   In other words, if someone has the right to a certain sort of treatment, others would be duty bound to respect that right. The broadest grounds for rights and duties are autonomy, beneficence, and justice.

Respect for autonomy – Respect for autonomy is the most fundamental of all moral principles. Three characteristics distinguish moral beings from other creatures and entitles them to special treatment:

> **1.** They have the ability to conceive of moral principles or rules.
>
> **2.** They have the ability to choose actions to conform with moral rules.
>
> **3.** They have the ability to limit actions to conform with those principles.

Having these abilities to be moral is essential to being an autonomous agent.   Autonomy, therefore, deserves ultimate respect because it is taken as the grounds for both moral treatment and moral responsibility. While it is clear that everyone is not fully autonomous, respect for autonomy requires that we presume autonomy and allow people to make their own choices, even when it seems that they are not doing what is best.

Truth telling – To make a choice, you must be aware of the facts that govern a situation, the alternatives, and the various implications. Respect for autonomy dictates that a physician tell a patient the truth, fully inform him of his condition, and list the available treatments so that the patient can make a decision about the future.

Beneficence – Beneficence instructs us to get involved and to do good for others (whether or not they want the good). Beneficence is a basic principle of ethics, derived from the understanding that if we need help, we want others to provide it. Since morality demands that we treat others as we wish to be treated (the golden rule), we are obliged to treat others with beneficence.

When we are able to help someone in need who rejects our help and instead wants to be left to "do his own thing," the principles of autonomy and beneficence collide. Deciding what to do becomes difficult. When we go ahead and act from beneficence and intentionally override or ignore another's autonomy, we are being paternalistic.

Beneficence versus autonomy – Since autonomy is the foundation of morality, we are inclined to respect an individual's choice, even when to us it appears to be a bad choice. However, there are situations in which beneficence trumps autonomy (e.g., we think we should interfere with the person poised to jump from a window ledge). Thus, we are left in need of a principle that would tell us when we must leave a person alone and when we must interfere for the good of another.

Autonomy-preserving paternalism – Immanuel Kant, an eighteenth-century philosopher who elevated the principle of autonomy within moral theory, has subtly provided such a tool in what can be called "the autonomy-preserving principle of paternalism." According to this principle, paternalistic interference can be justified if it creates, preserves, or restores autonomy. In other words, for the sake of maintaining endangered autonomy in the long run, we may override the immediate presumption of autonomy. But, the more severe and enduring the interference, the more physicians must question their own motivation and be concerned with the justification of their actions.

Beneficence directs the physician to help his patients with their health care needs and to act for their good. But when the patient refuses beneficial treatment, should it be forced upon him? Does it matter whether the patient is 51 years old or 15 years old? Will it matter whether the treatment is medication, blood transfusion, psychotherapy, or surgery? Should the likelihood of the procedure being successful make a difference?

Justice and fairness – Justice requires that we give each person his or her due; fairness demands that we treat people equally. Combined, they oblige us to treat similar differences in the same way. The traditional image of justice is the blindfolded figure of a woman holding a balance. She is the model of the distribution justice aims to achieve.

However, in the contemporary literature, John Rawls asks us to make decisions as if we were behind a "veil of ignorance." Rawls asks us to imagine that we are ignorant of our gender, race, health, age, social position, education, etc. From this position we are to formulate a general rule that would apply to all situations like the one we are considering. The decisions we make from such a hypothetically neutral stance would be just. And because they would be applicable to people in all similar situations, they would also be fair.

Justice and power – The question of justice is especially important in any relationship in which there is an imbalance of power such that one person is vulnerable to another. In the case of doctor and patient, the doctor's own ethics will ultimately affect the treatment of the patient; therefore, the doctor has a special obligation to consider what is due to the patient. Should the care provided reflect the patient's need, ability to pay, likelihood of benefit, or competing demands for treatment? The principle of justice may not always provide precise and definitive answers. However, it can help to eliminate some bad alternatives and to identify the most important considerations.

Special duties of physicians – Physicians have special duties, applying only to them, to employ their knowledge of science in treatment, to act to preserve health and life, and to do no harm. There are three possible sources for these special duties:

> **1.** The knowledge and skills that physicians acquire enables them to do what others cannot.
>
> **2.** Physicians traditionally take an oath that obligates them to satisfy the duties of their chosen profession.
>
> **3.** A contract with society gives physicians the exclusive right to practice medicine. This monopoly on medical practice is given with the understanding that the profession assumes the obligation for providing everyone who is in need with medical care.

Treat, preserve life, and do no harm – Physicians have the special obligations to treat, to preserve life, and to do no harm. These are the cornerstone principles of medical ethics that are embraced in the Hippocratic Oath. The first two obligations require the physician to render treatment and the third demands that the physician exercise caution and scientific judgment. Although the physician is obliged to conform with all three of these principles, sometimes the action required by one of them can conflict with the dictates of another. When these principles clash, there is no universal rule stating that one of these principles should override another. Whenever surgery is performed, we accept the fact that harm (e.g., infliction of pain and scars) is done for the sake of some other good (e.g., preserving life). Sometimes we reject the option of prolonging life because the necessary means would entail too great a harm (e.g., loss of function or infliction of pain). We may refuse to preserve lives because doing so would harm another (e.g., vital organs are not taken from someone who refuses consent). At times, there is no obviously better choice between alternatives and even the most paternalistic physician must accept the principle that the patient alone should be the one who decides whether life or harm should be chosen.

Physicians have the obligation to satisfy all of their general and special duties. However, it is often difficult to recognize them in clinical practice, and when they conflict, it is still more difficult to decide precisely what is the right thing to do. The interplay among the physician's several duties is both subtle and quite complex.

Autonomy and truth telling – Respect for the patient's autonomy requires "truth telling" by the physician. Patients need facts and having misinformation can lead to making different decisions. While there may be times when withholding the truth is justified, and there is always an issue of how much information constitutes truth telling, whenever the truth is sacrificed for reasons of beneficence, autonomy is diminished.

Medical ethics in medical education – During the course of medical education, there are two special moral issues that confront students: the use of animals and patients as research or teaching tools. Even though these are common features of the standard medical school curriculum, the thoughtful student must consider whether these practices are ethically justifiable.

Using animals for research and teaching – Peter Singer and Tom Reagan are primary advocates of animal rights who have argued that because animals can feel pain and can act to achieve goals, they are sufficiently like humans and should be treated with moral consideration. Therefore, when we would not do something to humans, we should also not do it to animals. If animal rights advocates are correct in their basic assumptions and arguments, animals should not be used as models in medical education, nor should they be used in research.

Animals differ from us is in that they cannot think or act in terms of moral principles and rules. If this characteristic is morally significant, perhaps there is a justification for treating humans and animals differently and it may be permissible to use animals in medical education and research. However, there would probably still be an ethical requirement for prudence, good treatment, and the avoidance of pain.

Using patients for research and teaching – In a hospital setting there are many experienced professionals available to provide patient care. Whenever a medical student or resident at the beginning of the learning curve performs a procedure that could be done more skillfully by someone with more experience, the learners and teachers are not acting for the good of the patient. The patient is subjected to greater risk of harm and discomfort; the learners and teachers are violating the dictum, "do no harm."

Furthermore, respect for autonomy requires us to avoid treating people merely as means to some end of our own, as tools for our own purposes. Taken together, these considerations suggest that patients should not be used in medical education.

Training programs must be morally acceptable – Reconsidering this issue from another perspective, it is clear that everyone needing medical attention would want to have trained and skilled physicians available to administer their care. Since medical education programs involving patients are the necessary means to achieving this desired expertise, such training programs must be morally acceptable. This confirmation does not, however, complete the picture of obligation. An ethical program of medical education must avoid harming patients and uphold all other obligations to them. Medical education has done an excellent job of protecting the health of patients, through attention to the selection of candidates, sequential learning, supervised practice, discussion, evaluation, and review.

Honesty with patients – Programs using patients in medical education must insist on clearly informing patients of the participation of students and residents in their treatment. Respect for patients requires more than a charming bedside manner; it demands that people be told the truth about who is being asked to do what for whom. Informing a patient of the student or resident status of the person who is providing treatment allows the patient both the opportunity to fulfill the moral duty of participation in the training project and the genuine pleasure of contributing to the training of a physician. This honesty also promotes the idea of patients as heroic partners engaged in the education of the community's future doctors.

Ethics in clinical practice – Every clinical case has its own unique features. In each situation, the right action must be determined. Sometimes this is easy, but often there are several conflicting moral demands and it is difficult to see what must be done. Examining a specific case will illustrate some of the typical complexities encountered in medical practice.

A case – Mr. R. had terminal cancer of the bowel with metastasis to his liver and lung. His family, in particular his son, had insisted to the private attending physician that the patient not be told that he had cancer and a fatal prognosis. Each day at rounds, the housestaff was confronted by the patient's questions: what was wrong with him, why he was continuing to lose weight, experiencing pain, and having difficulty holding down food. "Do I have cancer? Am I going to die?" he would ask. The housestaff fended off Mr. R.'s questions by saying that he should talk with his attending physician. Hampered and restricted in their care of the patient, they distanced themselves from him and were angry with both the family and attending physician for not allowing them to alleviate his legitimate worries.

Mr. R. had adequate judgment and he wanted to know the facts about his own condition. He knew that he was seriously ill, yet he was kept from the truth because of his family's wishes and his doctor's admonitions. These constraints on truth telling kept the housestaff and nursing staff from addressing the patient's worries and from being close to him during a time of suffering and concern. Although the plan against exposing the diagnosis was well intended, it removed the patient from the decision-making process, minimized his ability to manage his own illness and affairs, and deprived him of his autonomy. By not telling him the truth, the health care team also diminished its ability to provide an honest, close, supportive relationship with the hospital staff and failed to treat the patient justly. Truth telling has always been problematic in medicine. Regardless of prevailing social attitudes, a presumption in favor of truth telling is very strong. Truth telling in no way mitigates the physician's ongoing duty of benevolence that requires continued care and encouragement. "We will be with you, make you as pain-free as possible, and we will do everything we can for you." Such continued caring and reassurance for concerns about intractable pain and abandonment are essential aspects of the physician's role with the seriously and terminally ill. In an attempt to "protect" the patient and also to "protect" themselves, doctors who revert to distortion of the truth undermine the patient's autonomy, and at a deeper level, they risk the doctor/patient relationship. How the truth should be told to the patient may vary according to circumstances and customs, but the truth must be told if respect for the patient's autonomy is to be preserved.

Conclusion – Medical students and physicians must be aware of the ethical issues arising from the practice of medicine. With the ever-increasing pace of technology, the need for more service and greater access to medical care, all in the context of limited economic resources, the moral problems confronting physicians will multiply. Although doctors are not expected to be bioethicists, medicine cannot be practiced well without sensitivity to the moral dimension of patient care and without the competency to engage in moral reasoning and ethical decision making.

Sections of this chapter draw on material in a co-authored chapter, "Ethical Issues in Consultation-Liaison Psychiatry," by James Strain, Rosamond Rhodes, Daniel A. Moros, Bernard Baumrin forthcoming in *Medical Psychiatric Practice,* vol. 2, Alan Stoudemire, editor, American Psychiatric Press, Washington, D.C.

Chapter 14

A Summing Up of Ideas

• Be sure you have a personal study area where you can keep your books, notes, etc.

• As you study, jot down ideas, make a table, or graph data.

• Avoid creating jaundiced or psychedelic textbooks.

• Check your spelling for every word you aren't sure about, even in your own notes.

• Your most basic reference is a good medical dictionary.

• Making your own review tapes forces you to think about and organize information.

• Read through old exam questions even before you begin studying for a course to develop a sense of the content range, difficulty level, and amount of detail that you must achieve.

• The sheer volume of material that must be mastered in medical school far exceeds undergraduate demands.

• The level of detailed knowledge that is expected of medical students is vast.

• Cramming breeds confusion and forgetting and rarely leads to the level of mastery that is expected of medical students.

• It is important to have a study approach that will maximize long-term retention.

• A potentially damaging misconception is that an approach that works for another student will necessarily work for you.

• Read *The New England Journal of Medicine* every week.

• Read about every disease, patient, treatment, or condition that may be discussed, used as an example, or just mentioned in your classes in *Harrison's Principles of Internal Medicine.*

• You will need to understand the pH scale for expressing hydrogen ion concentration (acidity or basicity).

• Learn again what a mole is and what an equivalent is.

• An appreciation of the physical laws governing electricity including understanding the units of potential, current, and resistance are necessary for understanding the functioning of all cells and especially of nerves and muscles.

• You will discover that you must use logs (both base 10 and natural) quite often in your medical studies.

• Communicating is very important. It is especially important to be able to communicate effectively with your patients, often under circumstances where they are ill, frightened, don't wish to hear what you have to say, and are not especially knowledgeable about medicine.

• Practice explaining things to others every opportunity you get.

• Learn to take good notes.

• For the rest of your career you will need to find information so knowing how to use a library efficiently is very important.

• One of the most important factors to successful study is organizing and managing your time effectively.

• The most successful medical students take a highly organized approach to life.

• If you are in control of your time, you can afford to be spontaneous from time to time.

• Study groups provide a wealth of advantages.

- Take careful note of how your exams, study days, and important life commitments are spaced.

- Make a list of all important life maintenance activities that you must take care of on a weekly basis.

- Make a list of all leisure and social activities that you believe would be within reason to maintain while in medical school.

- It is likely that most weeks will follow a similar pattern, however, it is advisable to reconsider your plan at the start of each week.

- Like a new diet, an exercise program, or learning to drive a car, implementing a time-management plan can be a challenge.

- Make a study-life plan and stick to it.

- Find a regular place for study.

- Be completely up to date by the start of each new week.

- Don't forget that your spouse has a right to expect some time from you, too.

- Involve your children and your spouse in the construction of your time plan.

- Whenever a person takes action, the action performed could be either right or wrong.

- Medical decisions are serious moral matters.

- Feelings play an important role in right action.

- The virtuous person is virtuous both because she has principles and extends goodwill to everyone she meets.

- Caring feelings, along with attention to principles and theoretical analysis, are the requirements of morality.

- Whenever someone has a right, someone else has a duty.

• The good doctor will not look to her own interests but, to those of her patients, caring for them to promote their well-being.

• The good doctor will feel goodwill toward his patients, and from that feeling he will be able to give each patient what is morally due.

• Patients who are given good medical treatment may become upset or angry when they feel that their doctor does not care about them personally.

• Respect for autonomy is the most fundamental of all of the moral principles.

• To make a choice, a person must be aware of the facts that govern a situation, the alternatives, and the various implications.

• Beneficence instructs us to get involved and to do good for others (regardless of whether or not they want the good).

• Justice requires that we give each person his or her due; fairness demands that we treat people equally.

• Physicians have the special obligations to treat, to preserve life, and to do no harm.

• Respect for autonomy requires the physician to allow the patient to make his own decisions.

• Respect for patients requires more than a charming bedside manner; it demands that people be told the truth about who is being asked to do what for whom.

• Medicine cannot be practiced well without sensitivity to the moral dimension of patient care and without the competency to engage in moral reasoning and ethical decision making.

• Your challenge is to meet your new responsibilities with the least possible psychological stress.

• When a person views an event or situation as stressful, the body reacts by initiating the fight or flight response.

• Making your thoughts and attitudes self-supporting rather than self-defeating will help tremendously in succeeding in medical school.

• Put things into their proper perspective.

• Your medical school would not have accepted you if they did not feel you are capable of performing to their standards.

• View and treat other medical students as colleagues rather than as competitors.

• Medical school is not a competition; it is a time to get the best training you can, and to perform to your optimal level.

• Challenge yourself to create and live up to an appropriate standard of personhood and student performance.

• Study groups are stress relievers.

• Be preventive rather than reactive in problem solving.

• Getting needed help is not a sign of weakness, but of strength.

• Being a medical student will consume most of your time, energy, and attention.

• Try to keep completely up to date by studying the most recent material on a daily basis.

• Each week return to your time-management plan and fill in the content you expect to master each day to correspond with your course syllabi.

• Immediate review and memorization is the most time efficient way to study.